Maximize Your Medicare

Understanding Medicare,
Protecting Your Health,
And Minimizing Costs

Jae W. Oh, MBA, CLU® ChFC®

Copyright 2012 Jae W. Oh, MBA, CLU® ChFC®

Cover Art: Ani Cho Stone

Library of Congress Control Number: 2012515561

ISBN-13: 978-1480073425

ISBN-10: 1480073423

For my children

"I know everything that I need to know about Medicare."

-No one

How to Use This Book

Medicare is frequently misunderstood for many reasons. *Maximize Your Medicare* is intended to address these misunderstandings, so you can choose the right option for yourself. What you select will depend on the complicated combination of your medical situation, financial resources, family situation, and in the end, your mental outlook. This book may convince you that your situation is too complicated to decide for yourself. As a result, reading this book may encourage you to seek outside assistance. Even if this is your best option, this book will still be useful because it will help you ask informed questions, to make sure that you are being told all of the relevant facts.

Ultimately, this book wants to help you avoid this well-known conversation:
Q. "Why didn't you tell me?"
A. "You didn't ask."

The book explains original Medicare and the enrollment timeline. *Maximize Your Medicare* informs you of the important dates, how those dates relate to you, what to do, and when. There are many exceptions to these rules, and perhaps surprisingly, many are in your favor. *Maximize Your Medicare* points out some examples of exceptions, so that you know about certain things that you must keep in mind.

The book contains many examples of real-life situations. They are called *"This Happens."* They are real-life examples (the names have been removed).

Here is a quick sample:

This happens.

When a married couple has one newly Medicare-eligible person, and one who is not Medicare-eligible, both covered by a group health insurance plan, it can become quite complicated. Choosing wrongly can be very, very costly. "Choosing wrongly" can also mean staying with the status quo. Do not misunderstand: doing nothing is making a conscious choice. An extra layer of complexity is introduced if one spouse has medical conditions, or requires constant medical attention. There cannot be one answer because group plans differ greatly depending on the employer as well as the insurance company offering the group insurance.

This happens.

This book will point out factors which should be used in making a decision. While the situations presented cannot possibly be exactly like yours, they are meant with one message in mind: you are not alone, and there is always a way to choose amongst a seemingly dizzying number of options. *Maximize Your Medicare* sets out to help you do just that.

Medicare is constantly evolving, and it will continue to do so. *Maximize Your Medicare* will evolve with it. You can go to the website www.maximizeyourmedicare.com to find updates, corrections and additional examples of "*This happens.*" Future updates to this book will be available when Medicare announces premiums for 2013. *Upon examination of the Medicare Advantage plans announced for 2013, it appears that the premiums, copays and coinsurance terms will worsen for Medicare beneficiaries, not only for Medicare Advantage beneficiaries, but for all Medicare beneficiaries due to worsening cost sharing terms of Medicare Part A and Medicare Part B.* If you have purchased this book, in physical or electronic form (eBook), then you can register for the site and then receive your updates free of charge.

The conclusions of this book are the informed opinions of the author. They are not endorsed by, nor do they represent the opinions of any insurance company or any other party. Nothing in this book should be construed to be an offer or advice to purchase a particular policy from any particular company.

The facts upon which these opinions are given are subject to change or error. These facts can and should be checked by the reader or advisor. If you have questions, you should seek professional advice.

Two pieces of advice for using this book: First, read the Glossary at the end. Some of the terms may apply to you. Some of the terms may be new to you. That way, you can notice language in this book, in your description of benefits, or in conversations with professionals. Don't let the jargon get in the way of you protecting yourself. Second, don't skim this book: it isn't designed to be 500 pages long. That is intentional. There is valuable information that you may be able to use, in every section.

Introduction

Why All the Fuss About Medicare?

In 2013, 9,200 people will turn 65, EVERY DAY. According to the U.S. Census Bureau (2008), that is approximately the number of people that are becoming entitled to Medicare every single day. The baby boomers have arrived. It is virtually guaranteed that you know someone whose life is affected by Medicare.

Complaints about various aspects of Medicare are everywhere, but let's step back for a moment. If you are 63 years old, private health insurance costs approximately $400-$500 a month (it can be much more if you choose very comprehensive coverage). In addition to the $400-$500 monthly premium, the deductible amount is generally $2,500, if not more than that. For those that are seriously ill, and assuming that insurance is available at all, premiums alone can approach $1,000 a month. If you want to add medications on top of that you're talking about another hundred dollars a month, plus copays. As those with extensive medications can tell you, prescriptions can be $300-400 a month. Your maximum annual out-of-pocket expenses can approach $10,000 a year, in addition to the premiums. That is your situation just prior to Medicare eligibility.

Under Medicare, let's take a look at your total costs. For most people, original Medicare (Medicare Part A and Medicare Part B) costs about a hundred dollars ($104.90 for 2013, or more if your income exceeds $85,000). Additionally, a 65-year old can purchase a policy, with no network, no deductible, and no concept of annual out-of-pocket maximum (because coinsurance will be $0), for about $175 a month. The two premiums (Medicare Part B and Medigap) define your entire medical cost (not including prescriptions).

Prescription coverage under Medicare receives attention in the press, but it is usually due to the confusion regarding the Coverage Gap (known as the "donut hole"), and the fact that people cannot believe the cost of an individual medication. For 2013, the national average for stand-alone prescription drug plans (Medicare Part D) is $30.18 a month. Even if you took the most expensive medications available, the maximum amount of medications would be, at most, $400 a month. That includes the period in which you experienced the infamous coverage gap ("donut hole").

The total costs? Even if you went all the way through the donut hole, for the same $500-$700 a month you could get the same type of the same price as you received before Medicare, but you would have perfect insurance (except in the most extreme cases). These are the real facts: there is no getting around these numbers. For people that have been living with an incurable disease, the savings under Medicare will be $10,000 a year. That's right, $10,000 a year (and more) is being saved by people with serious medical conditions under Medicare.

In other words, Medicare, coupled with the right plan for the individual situation, is superior to the coverage that you can obtain in the private (or group) market before the time you were eligible for Medicare. It is both cheaper and more comprehensive. By cheaper, it is commonly $5,000 a year less expensive. By more comprehensive, your out-of-pocket expenses will most likely be lower, and in a serious medical situation, the out-of-pocket expenses will be dramatically lower. Medicare can literally keep a household out of bankruptcy.

Some may say "Well, I only pay $300 a month." That is because someone else (an employer or the younger employees in the group) is subsidizing you. It has nothing to do with Medicare. NOTHING.

These are not aggressive estimates. They are real-life, market-relevant numbers. If anything, I would say that Medicare beneficiaries should want Medicare to stay in its existing state, and to not weaken further from here.

Aye, there's the rub. If you watch the national news for about five minutes (at most), you will hear talk about Medicare. You will hear talk about the fact that the Medicare system may be insolvent in the future, or that the Medicare system may be overhauled in a very fundamental way. If that occurs, then the choices that I will present may become unavailable. Substantial restructuring of Medicare is the outcome that should worry you.

When you think about the fact that Medicare can change, and largely for the worse, then you can understand the number #1 recommendation of this book:

Get the best coverage that you can reasonably afford, while you can, because your choices are probably going to worsen, due to your age, declining health, and changing Medicare system.

All three of the factors above (age, health, changing Medicare system) are going in the same direction: away from you. The only question is when, not if, this will (most likely) occur. If you do nothing, if you don't get as complete information as you can, then you are taking an enormous risk, whether you know it or not. It is fine to accept risk because consequences (which can be beyond your control) have dictated that to you. That is beyond the scope of this short book. This book reveals the risks you may be taking, risks that you didn't know you were taking. You can find my recommendation on which risks you can (and should) avoid.

There is the age-old cliché that says that "you hope for the best and plan for the worst." Medical insurance under original Medicare, when combined with a Medigap policy (also known as Medicare supplemental insurance, a Medicare supplement), allows you to do this. You can largely protect against the most likely expense you will encounter as you naturally age, the most likely expense to cause you and your spouse/family worry, and the most likely source of financial distress to you and your extended family. I hope that this book will be of some use to you. But before we dive into the details, we need to get one thing straight.

Let's Get One Thing Straight

Health insurance is not the same thing as auto insurance or homeowner's insurance. Nevertheless, this is the kind of comparison that you can hear in every coffee shop, in every corner of the nation. Comparing health insurance to auto insurance is like comparing apples to oranges. They are both a type of fruit, and that is where the similarity ends. It is a fundamentally incorrect comparison to make. Why?

Say you get in a car accident, and you completely wreck your car, but walk away unscathed. What is the cost to you? Do you know? Absolutely. Open a Kelley Blue Book, and you will be able to determine the salvage value of your car within hundreds of dollars. You can replace your car with an almost-exact copy.

On the other hand, imagine that you become seriously ill, and are diagnosed with a disease. What are your costs then? Can you speculate on the price of recovery? You cannot predict when those costs will cease. You cannot predict if you can go back to work in order to repay those new, unknown costs. You cannot calculate it, and your error rate can be in the tens of thousands of dollars. The cost can bankrupt your household, and the outstanding liability will make you indebted to the government for the remainder of your life. In other words, the downside of not protecting yourself in case you become seriously ill is many, many, many times worse than getting into a car accident. You cannot estimate the maximum loss of money, time, and well-being if you become ill. And the older your get, the more extreme it becomes, because the likelihood of becoming seriously ill is greater.

When you compare this outcome to the effort it takes to become knowledgeable about Medicare and the implications of the decisions you make, it should be obvious that reading on will be worth the time. Maybe I am wrong. Probably not.

Chapter 1 - Enrollment in Medicare

Medicare Initial Enrollment

What I'm going to do at this time is discuss the Medicare eligibility timeline. There are many different dates moving around, confusing terms with respect to eligibility, when to sign up, when there are penalties, and when there are not. I will start with the base case.

The base case: the initial Medicare Part A and Medicare Part B eligibility date will be the first day of the month that you turn 65 years old. This is the first date that you can be covered under Medicare Part A and Medicare Part B.

For example, let's use the name listed on the card, Jane Doe. If Jane was born on February 13, 1948, then her first date of Medicare eligibility will be February 1, 2013.

There is an exception to this rule, which occurs for those born on the first day of any month. If Jane was born on February 1, 1948, for example, the first date of Medicare eligibility is actually going to be the first date of the prior month. In this case, Jane's first date of Medicare eligibility will be January 1, 2013.

Signing up for Medicare Part A and Part B is usually quite a simple matter. If you are already receiving Social Security or RRB (Railroad Retirement Board) benefits when you turn 65 years old, then you will automatically get your Medicare card, the well-known red, white, and blue card with first date of eligibility printed right on it for you. That will be the case if you have been receiving Social Security payments prior to the age of 65.

It looks like this:

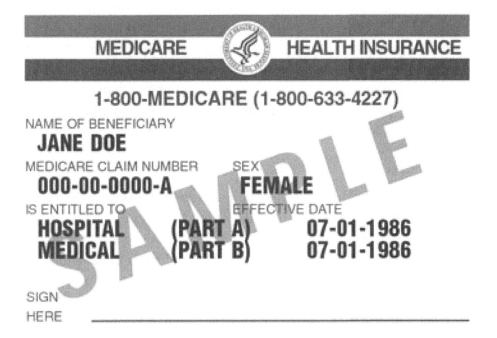

For Jane Doe, let's continue to use the February 13, 1948 as Jane's birthday. In this case, the first date that she can enroll is November 1, 2012, which is three months prior to her initial eligibility date. That is the first date that she can sign up for Medicare; her effective date will not be until February 1, 2013.

You can choose to not enroll in Medicare Part B until three months after the month that you turn 65 years old, and face no penalty. Let's return to Jane. She turns 65 years old in February. Add three months to that. Jane can enroll in Medicare all the way up until May 31, 2013 without penalty. This is commonly known as the Medicare Initial Enrollment Period.

Very important note: if you wait until the month of your 65 birthday, or later, then your Medicare Part B effective date will be delayed. Even though Jane Doe can sign up during February,

14

March April and May, her first date of coverage will be delayed. If Jane signed up in February, the first date of coverage would be March 1. If Jane signed up in March, then the first date of coverage would be May 1. If Jane signed up in April, then the first date of coverage would be July 1. Lastly, if Jane signed up in May, then the first date of coverage would be August. Confused? The easiest solution: enroll during the month prior to your first possible eligibility date AT THE LATEST.

Late Enrollment Penalty

Let's now consider the case if you decide to not enroll in Medicare Part B during the Medicare Initial Enrollment Period. Back to Jane Doe, who was born on February 13, 1948. Now, say it is August 15, 2013. Beginning in June, Jane Doe will pay a penalty for every year that she does not enroll in Medicare Part B. You might think that she could've simply signed up, and Medicare Part B would be effective September 1, 2013, right? Wrong.

When you do not enroll in Medicare Part B during the Medicare Initial Enrollment Period, and have no "creditable coverage" (meaning that you have health insurance certified by the Medicare system), then the next time that you will be allowed to enroll is called the General Election Period (GEP), which runs from the beginning of January through the end of March every year. Your first effective date of coverage under Medicare will be July 1 of that year.

Once you are a penalty-paying beneficiary, then your first effective date of coverage under Medicare can only be January or July. You will need to check with your Social Security office in order to confirm the first date that Medicare Part B will be effective. To make matters worse, you would be charged a rate that includes a penalty for not enrolling during your Medicare Initial Enrollment Period.

Group Insurance and Part B Enrollment

Some group employer plans require that you enroll in Medicare Part B. Some do not. Do not rely on others to confirm this information. Confirm it yourself by locating the language in the Summary of Benefits of the employer-sponsored plan. Sometimes, human resource departments do not spell this out for you clearly. When you contact your human resources or employee benefit department, ask the human resources person to point out the location where the language exists in the Summary of Benefits that explains the requirement to enroll in Medicare Part B. *Sometimes, human resources personnel get it wrong themselves.* While you can blame the human resources department for their ineptitude, the one paying the higher cost will be... you. It is highly unlikely (good luck) that you will have any recourse to your (former) employer if the HR department neglects to inform you.

Enrollment Before 65 (Disability, ESRD, ALS)

There are certain situations in which you can be eligible for Medicare prior to the age of 65. For example, if you have end stage renal disease (ESRD), or if you have received 24 consecutive months of Social Security disability benefits, then you may be eligible for early enrollment into Medicare. The issue is obtaining Social Security disability benefits. That is a very difficult task. You may know someone in this situation; it is not simple. There are usually lawyers and court dates involved (there are Social Security attorneys). If you have ESRD, please refer to the Glossary for a very important fact about renal disease patients.

However, if you are awarded Social Security disability benefits, then you will be automatically enrolled into Medicare Part A and Medicare Part B after 24 consecutive months of receiving Social Security disability payments. On the first day of the third year that you receive Social Security disability benefits, you will be automatically enrolled in Medicare Part A, and will be eligible for

Medicare Part B. Depending on your net worth and income, you may also be eligible for the Low Income Subsidy (LIS, also known as the "Extra Help" program) at that time. There is more information regarding the LIS is contained in Chapter 5.

ALS (Lou Gehrig's Disease) patients are eligible for both Medicare Part A and Medicare Part B automatically on the month that disability benefits begin.

One thing to note: military disability is not the same thing as Social Security disability. For example, there is no such thing as partial Social Security disability, as there is under the rules established by the Veterans Administration. In addition, the process of obtaining VA disability benefits is entirely different from the process of applying for Social Security disability benefits.

You May Not Qualify At All

Unfortunately there is a situation where you cannot qualify for Medicare Part A or Part B. That is your situation if you and your spouse have not paid Social Security taxes for the required amount of time, which is 40 quarters. If you are in doubt, then you need to contact your local Social Security office or the Social Security website (www.socialsecurity.gov).

Chapter 2. Medicare Part A (Hospital Insurance)

Let's start with Medicare Part A. Medicare Part A can be thought of as coverage for the cost of facilities. A summary of the charges for Medicare Part A are provided in Table 1 at the end of this chapter (source: www.Medicare.gov). Please make sure that you know and understand the definition of the terms *deductible* and *copays* before proceeding. They can be found in the Glossary.

Hospital Inpatient Stay

Deductible: $1184 per benefit period
First 60 Days Cost: You pay $0. Medicare pays.
Days 61-100 Cost: You pay $296 a day. Medicare pays the rest.
Days 101-150 Cost: You pay $592 a day. Medicare pays the rest.
Days 150+ Cost: You pay 100%

Skilled Nursing Facility Care Stay

First 20 Days Cost: You pay $0. Medicare pays.
Days 21-100 Cost: You pay the first $148 a day. Medicare pays the rest.
Days 100+: You pay 100%
ONLY after a 3-day inpatient stay at a hospital
Skilled Nursing Care is a technical term and does not include solely custodial care.

Inpatient Psychiatric Care

190 days lifetime benefit, Medicare pays 100%

Hospice Care

You pay:
$0 for hospice care
A copayment of up to $5 per prescription for outpatient prescription drugs for pain and symptom management
5% of the Medicare-allowed charge for inpatient respite care (short-term care given by another caregiver, so the usual caregiver can rest)
Medicare doesn't cover room and board when you get hospice care in your home or another facility where you live (like a nursing home).

Blood

In most cases, the hospital gets blood from a blood bank at no charge, and you won't have to pay for it or replace it. If the hospital has to buy blood for you, you must either pay the hospital costs for the first 3 units of blood you get in a calendar year or have the blood donated.

Premium

The good news, of course, is that the price is zero. If you do not qualify for Medicare Part A, however, then you face very large costs. You can purchase Medicare Part A at a price of $451 a month, and a 10% Late Enrollment Penalty, which lasts twice as long as the period in which you did not sign up, but were eligible, if you enroll after the Medicare Initial Election Period (open enrollment period) ends.

How long do you pay this penalty? You pay the penalty for twice as long as the period that you did not enroll. An example would be easier. If you delay for 3 years, then your penalty would be 10% per year for 3 x 2 = 6 years.

Deductibles

The negatives are that there are large deductibles associated with Medicare Part A. The largest of these is the deductible that accompanies a hospital stay. For a hospital stay in 2013, the deductible is $1184. For every benefit period (see Key Term: Benefit Period in the next section), you are obligated to pay the first $1184 of total hospital costs. The table above shows the schedule of deductibles that you are obligated to pay if you are admitted to a hospital.

The very high deductibles and copayments required under Medicare Part A are the primary reason that being covered solely by original Medicare (Part A and Part B) is a very bad idea, and should be avoided, if at all possible. Any Medicare Advantage or Medigap plan, with prescription drug coverage, will be superior, and potentially save you thousands of dollars if you are admitted even once to a hospital in any given year. If you or someone you know is in extreme financial distress, then there is governmental assistance available under the LIS ("Limited Income Subsidy") or the "Extra Help" program. Finally, there are MA plans with no premium, which have all been approved by the CMS.

In addition to the high cost of deductibles and copays that accompany Medicare Part A, one other consideration is that the amounts of these deductibles and copays are determined by Medicare. They are subject to change annually. They are the source of annual debate and speculation. You don't need a crystal ball in order to predict which direction these amounts are going over time: up. It is a very large concern that the Medicare system itself is experiencing extreme fiscal stress; one way to "fix it?" Raise taxes. Another way? Raise deductibles and copays. Given these alternatives, the best solution is to obtain a policy to cover these potential out-of-pocket expenses.

Copays

Copays that accompany Medicare Part A are also very, very expensive. For example, if you require a hospital admission, then after you have been charged the first $1184, which is the deductible, there will be copays as well.

If you need to stay at a hospital for longer than 60 days, the daily amount that you would pay with Medicare Part A will be $296. It gets worse, and can be $592 a day between days 101-150. Beyond that, you are responsible for 100% of the daily cost.

Key Term: Benefit Period

The key term to know about the Medicare Part A is "benefit period." The Medicare Part A deductible for hospital stays is not an annual deductible. It is a deductible which exists for each benefit period. The benefit period can best be understood as a medical episode. For example, if you have a right knee joint replacement in January, then you may be admitted to a hospital. Then, you will require rehabilitation, which may be done at home, or at a facility.

Six months later, imagine that your other knee requires joint replacement surgery. This is a new benefit period. Strictly speaking, the benefit period expires 60 calendar days after being discharged from the hospital for that particular medical issue. If you have a different medical problem that requires hospitalization within that 60 days, or if you are readmitted to the hospital for the same issue after 60 calendar days, then that is another benefit period. You will owe another $1184, and you may repeat this for an unlimited number of times in one calendar year.

Now, it is highly unlikely that you will have many different benefit periods in a year. Requiring five separate hospital admissions within one calendar year is pretty bad fortune for a person, to say the least. However, it illustrates the fact that the deductible is not the deductible that you normally presume. If you or someone you know has been admitted to a hospital and has seen an itemized bill can confirm, it is very common that the cost of a single hospital stay will exceed the deductible; that means that you will most likely have to pay the entire deductible amount per hospital admission.

Skilled Nursing Care Facilities

Consider skilled nursing care facilities under Medicare. If you review the list at the beginning of this chapter, you can see that the first 20 days at a skilled nursing care facility are paid by Medicare. Between days 20-100, you will have to pay coinsurance, which is the first $148 per day. Medicare will pay the remainder. This amount is set annually, and may (almost certainly will) increase in the future. Medicare will pay for the remainder.

Since most skilled nursing home facilities cost more than $200/day, you will be most likely have to pay the entire $148 per day for days 21-40 of a stay at a skilled nursing care facility. This type of care does not include custodial care, which is the care required for completing tasks such as doing groceries, and cooking.

A major change was introduced during November 2012. In the past, you were required to be making progress towards recovery in order to be eligible for Medicare benefits. However, this is no longer the case. You can be in maintenance status at a skilled nursing facility, and still receive Part A benefits. For persons that have suffered a stroke, or have been afflicted with Alzheimer's disease, this is a very welcome change.

It is unclear at this point whether or not you can be admitted to a hospital under "observation status," and then be transferred to a skilled Nursing Care Facility under maintenance status, and receive Medicare Part A benefits. In the past, this has been a controversial issue. First, you must understand the meaning of the complicated term "observation status."

Observation Status

When you are admitted to the hospital, you may or may not know that you can be admitted as inpatient or under observation status. If you look at Table 1, Medicare Part A Cost Sharing, then you will note that under Medicare Part A, the cost of a Skilled Nursing Facility occurs ONLY after a 3-day stay. However, if you are placed under observation status, this DOES NOT QUALIFY. If you then go to a skilled nursing care facility, you will be responsible for the entire cost. It is not covered by Medicare Part A, Medicare Advantage (Medicare Part C), or Medigap. It is very important that you know whether or not you have been admitted inpatient or under observation status. Otherwise, you could face very expensive costs, and worse than that, it may come as a total surprise.

Table 1. Medicare Part A Cost Sharing (2013)

Source: CMS

Hospital Inpatient stay	First 60 Days Cost: You pay $0. Days 61 - 100: You pay the first $296 a day. Medicare pays the rest. Days 101 – 150: You pay the first $592 a day. Medicare pays the rest. Days 150 +: You pay 100%	Deductible: $1184 per benefit period (See Glossary for definition of benefit period)
Skilled Nursing Facility Care Stay	First 20 Days Cost: Medicare pays 100% Days 20-100: You pay the first $148 a day; Medicare pays for the remainder. Days 101+: You pay 100%	ONLY after a 3-day inpatient stay at a hospital Skilled Nursing Care is a technical term and does not include solely custodial care.
Inpatient Psychiatric Care	190 days lifetime benefit, Medicare pays 100% You pay $0.	

Chapter 3. Medicare Part B (Medical Insurance)

Premium

Let's move to Medicare Part B. It is called medical insurance by the CMS (Centers for Medicare & Medicaid Services), but I would've called it services. Premiums are indexed to income, which means that if you earn more than $85,000 as an individual, or greater than $170,000 filing jointly, you can be charged more for your Part B. You will be charged according to the schedule in Table 2 (source: www.Medicare.gov/cost).

In many cases, this amount is deducted directly from your Social Security check. This is not a requirement. That is, you can receive a bill for the monthly premium if you so choose. In some cases, direct bill is the only possible way to pay. For example, federal employees do not generally receive a Social Security check. In addition, you may have saved money in a tax-advantaged savings account. For example, a little known fact is that funds in an HSA (Health Savings Account) can be used to pay for your Medicare Part B premium.

Annual Deductible

In addition to the monthly premium, there is an annual deductible, which is known as the Part B deductible. For 2013, this amount is $147 per calendar year. You are obligated to pay the first $147 for medical services received. Due to the Patient Protection and Affordable Care Act (PPACA), a fee cannot to be charged to you for your annual preventive care checkup. In other words, the preventative care screening is complimentary and you should not be charged.

There are a few important points here to keep in mind. First, all services you receive must be deemed to be reasonable and necessary by the medical provider. Medicare, and any plan in addition to Medicare, will require this before paying any benefits. Hint: before receiving a diagnostic exam or therapy, simply ask the person if that exam or therapy is medically necessary. A confident, competent medical professional should not be offended by this question. If a medical professional becomes defensive when asked this, then you need to ask yourself some serious questions. Second, the $147 is based on Medicare's allowed charges. Allowed charges are discussed just below. So, if a service received has an allowed charge of $100, and the doctor charges you $120, only $100 counts towards the deductible. Third, the deductible is defined by the Medicare on an annual basis. The entire cost sharing arrangement under Medicare is changed by the government every year. That means that it can move up or down every year.

That is a consistent theme of this book; the Medicare system can change, and it is most likely to change for the worse in the long run. Before it does, you should use the options at your disposal to secure your healthcare coverage, while you are able to do so. Once limits are imposed by the Medicare system, then these options may not be available. You are putting your faith in a government-controlled program. This is much too important for you to leave it in anyone else's hands other than your own.

Coinsurance

Once you have paid the $147 annual deductible, then you have the coinsurance arrangement with the Medicare system. The Medicare system will pay for 80% of approved, medically necessary services. You will be obligated to pay for the remaining 20%. If you require surgery, and the physician charges $30,000, then you will owe at least $6,000. Hold on a second. Could you owe more than $6,000, when that is 20% of the total cost? Yes. You can owe more than this. It is very important to understand what this 80% and 20% means. Medicare will pay 80% of the Medicare-allowed charge. What is the Medicare-allowed charge?

Key Term: Medicare-Allowed Charge

Medicare has a long list and extensive, almost exhaustive, list of services and treatments delivered by doctors or medical professionals. Each item has an amount which it will pay to medical providers for that particular service. That is the Medicare-allowed charge. Presuming that the service is deemed reasonable and necessary, Medicare will pay 80% of the allowed charge, leaving you with 20% as an out-of-pocket expense.

Confusion often occurs when the doctor/medical provider charges more than the Medicare-allowed charge. A medical provider can bill up to 15% more than the Medicare-allowed charge. When this the case, then a number of different scenarios can occur. First, the doctor may accept the Medicare-allowed charge as full payment. You will simply owe the 20% of the Medicare-allowed charge. However, the medical provider may not accept the Medicare-allowed charge as full payment. So, in addition to the 20% of the Medicare-allowed charge that the Medicare system does not pay (which you will have to pay), you will also have to pay the entire extra amount that the medical provider charges above and beyond the Medicare-allowed charge. The amount above the Medicare-allowed charge is called the Medicare Part B Excess. Confused? Let's try an example to illustrate this important concept. It is important because then you can make a better-informed decision to Maximize Your Medicare.

Part B Excess Example

> ### *This happens.*
>
> A doctor wants to charge $30,000 for some procedure and the Medicare-allowed charge is $27,000. In addition, I will also presume that you have already satisfied the $147 annual Part B deductible. In this case, the doctor can choose to take the $27,000 and accept that as full payment. In this case, the physician has accepted the Medicare "allowed charge."
>
> However, the doctor can also send you the entire bill. What will happen is Medicare will pay for 80% of $27,000 (which 80% x $27,000 = $21,600), and you will have to pay $5,400 (=20% of $27,000). In addition, you will need to pay the entire amount that the doctor charges that is above the Medicare "allowed charge" amount. In this example, that is $3,000 ($30,000 less $27,000). Therefore, your out-of-pocket expenses would be $5,400 + $3,000 = $8,400.
>
> Total Bill = $30,000.
>
> Medicare-allowed charge= $27,000.
>
> Medicare Pays = $27,000 x 80% = $21,600, NOT $30,000 x 80%.
>
> You Pay 20% of Medicare-allowed charge: $27,000 - $21,600 = $5,400.
>
> You Pay the Entire Part B Excess Charge = $30,000 - $27,000 = $3,000.
>
> Your Total Cost = $5,400 + $3,000 = $8,400.
>
> *This happens.*

The fact is that the surgeon is entitled to charge this amount within the existing rules of Medicare. If you have to pay for the Medicare Part B Excess even once in your lifetime on this type of procedure, then you might guess that the extra premium paid would have more than paid for this risk by a very wide margin.

It is important to note that under almost every group plan, employer-provided plan, as well as under every Medicare Advantage (MA) plan (including MAPD), the Part B Excess is not covered. While the probability may be small, the potential financial effect can be dramatic. You need to carefully consider this point when deciding on the proper coverage under Medicare. The benefit of having this paid, without worry, may be worth the extra cost. This is particularly true for those that have known medical issues when entering the Medicare Initial Enrollment Period. Under the existing Medicare system, only Medigap Plan F, High-Deductible Plan F, and Plan G cover the Part B Excess Charge. In addition, one type of MA, called PFFS, can result in no Part B Excess Charge.

Cancelling Medicare Part B

Cancelling Medicare Part B is a serious matter, but you can do it. You will need to go to your local Social Security Administration office itself, and go through an interview. That will allow you to fill in a form named CMS-1763. The SSA will not mail you one, and it is not available online. The reason is that if you attempt to re-enroll, then you may be required to pay a penalty. Then again, if you are cancelling Medicare Part B to enter into another plan which is deemed to be creditable coverage, then you can re-enter Medicare Part B without penalty. The SSA wants to make sure that you understand the consequences. This is the "deep end of the pool," and needs to be handed carefully.

Table 2. Medicare Part B Cost Sharing (2013)

Source: CMS

Individual	Joint	Monthly Premium
$85,000 or less	$170,000 or less	$104.90
$85,001 - $107,000	$170,001 - $214,000	$146.90
$107,001 - $160,000	$214,001 - $320,000	$209.80
$160,001 - $214,000	$320,000 - $428,000	$272.70
Greater than $214,000	Greater than $428,000	$335.70

Chapter 4. Medicare Part C (Medicare Advantage)

Let's turn attention to Medicare Part C, more commonly known as Medicare Advantage. It actually replaces your red, white, and blue Medicare card. That said, you still need to pay the Medicare Part B monthly premium of $104.90. A Medicare Advantage plan must cover at least what Medicare covers (regulated by law). There are many different types of Medicare Advantage (also known as MA) plans. You have received, or you will receive many, many advertisements via mail regarding MA plans. You can also see the available plans in your area on http://www.medicare.gov.

Medicare Advantage Plans

There are a dizzying number of different types of Medicare Advantage plans. Frequently, the same insurance company will offer clients multiple options. Please know that this book will refer to the entire set as Medicare Advantage or MA. This includes plans in which prescription drug coverage is included, known as Medicare Advantage Prescription Drug plans (MAPD).

Here are the different types of Medicare Advantage plans:

* HMO (Health Maintenance Organization)

* PPO (Preferred Provider Organization)

* PFFS (Private Fee-for-Service)

* POS (Point of Service)

* HMO-SNP (Special Needs Plan)

Each type of Medicare Advantage will differ slightly, and each has some distinctive characteristics.

Health Maintenance Organization (HMO): You will need to specify a Primary Care Physician (PCP), who will refer you to specialists as necessary. All providers must be in the network. If you obtain routine medical care for out-of-network medical providers, neither Medicare or the HMO will pay any benefits, and you will be responsible for the entire cost. HMOs can be offered with and without prescription drug benefits. In some states, there is a partial rebate of the Medicare Part B premium that accompanies your participation in certain HMOs.

Preferred Provider Organization (PPO): You do not need to select a Primary Care Physician. You can seek medical services from providers outside the network, but with a different, higher cost sharing arrangement. Generally, the number of medical providers that accept a PPO is greater than the number that accepts an HMO (of the same insurance company). Prescription drug benefits are frequently included in these plans.

Private Fee-for-Service (PFFS): You can use a medical provider of your choice, but that provider must accept Medicare assignment of benefits, which means that it must accept Medicare's allowed charge as full payment. As a result, there is no possibility of Part B Excess Charge under this plan. However, a provider has the choice to accept you on a case-by-case basis, except in emergencies. This means that if you go to a doctor for one illness, and you are accepted, that does not guarantee that the same doctor must accept you the next time you attempt to receive services from that medical provider. PFFS plans may, or may not, include prescription drug benefits. PFFS is the only Medicare Advantage plan in which you can purchase a separate, stand-alone prescription drug plan (Part D). Lastly, if you attempt to cancel your PFFS by using a Special Election Period (SEP), you must request permission in order to do so.

Point of Service (POS): You will need to specify a Primary Care Physician (PCP), who will refer you to specialists as necessary. If you seek medical attention from those inside the network, then your PCP will coordinate benefits and administer the cost sharing terms as a courtesy to you. If you seek medical attention from those outside the network, you will be required to file claims, send in bills, etc by yourself. You will be required to code your own claims in accordance with the Centers for Medicare & Medicaid Services.

HMO-SNP (Special Needs Plan): There are three general types of HMO-SNPs. The first is when you have a chronic illness. The second is when you are resident in a skilled nursing facility. The third is when you qualify for both Medicare and Medicaid. You must qualify to enroll for these plans. You will need to select a primary care physician (PCP), and depending on the SNP, there will be specific types of formularies for your particular chronic illness, if that is the basis of acceptance to the HMO-SNP.

You will almost certainly need to have a case worker assigned to you by the Department of Health and Human Services and the Social Security Administration. In addition, an insurance company will most likely appoint its own individual assistant in order to coordinate benefits. The level of assistance granted is extremely complicated, and depends on your net worth and income. If you qualify, then the monthly premium is usually zero.

All medical services must administered by providers in the HMO's network. If you receive services from a non-network provider, then you must pay the entire bill. Medicare will not pay and your HMO-SNP will also not pay.

Medicare Advantage Prescription Drug (MAPD) Plans

Medicare Advantage Prescription Drug Plans combine health insurance with prescription drug coverage in one plan. Some of the different types of Medicare Advantage plans listed in the previous section can also be an MAPD. For example, a Medicare Advantage plan, which is also an HMO, may or may not include prescription coverage.

Important fact: If you have an MA or an MAPD plan, you cannot have a separate, additional stand-alone Prescription Drug Plan (Part D). The exception to this is PFFS, in which case you can have a separate PDP, or in certain cases, prescription drug benefits are embedded in the PFFS plan itself. If you elect a Medicare Advantage that does not include prescription benefits that is ruled as creditable coverage by the Medicare system, then you must have another source by which to defray prescription costs if you're on medications, or you will have to pay for prescriptions entirely from your own funds. In addition to this, you will be subject to the enrollment penalty at the time that you do enroll in a stand-alone Medicare Part D (prescription drug plan), or a Medicare Advantage plan that does include prescription benefits. For those that receive discount prescriptions through the Veterans Administration, it may be acceptable to select an MA without a prescription plan. That is up to you, and you should compare the out-of-pocket prescription costs under an MAPD, and compare it to the costs paid through the VA. It is likely that the VA is superior with respect to price given that the premium is zero, with the exception of insulin (more on this later). Some veterans prefer to obtain their prescriptions from a local pharmacy, and therefore, they choose an MAPD or a stand-alone prescription drug plan.

Medicare Advantage Initial Enrollment

The first date that you can enroll for a Medicare Advantage is the same as if you are enrolling in Medicare Part B. All of the exceptions also apply, from early qualification to Special Election Period (SEP). This will also be the same date on which you can initially enroll in Medicare Part B, and Medicare Part D, a stand-alone prescription drug plan (PDP).

Let's go back to Jane Doe, born on February 13, 1948.

In this example, November 1, 2012 is the first date she can enroll in MA/MAPD, or Part D, and the last date that she can enroll will be May 31, 2013. In short, the same rules apply to Medicare Advantage plans as well as to Medicare Part B and Medicare Part D. If she does not enroll in Medicare Part B and Part D between these dates, she will only be able to sign up during the General Election Period (GEP), unless she qualifies for a special situation, a Special Election Period (SEP).

If Jane does not qualify for a SEP, then she will have the Part D penalty as described in Chapter 5. If she chooses to not enroll in a Medicare Advantage plan but does accept just Medicare Part A and Part B, then there will be no Part B penalty, but she will be subject to the Part D penalty. The bottom line: if you enroll late, then you will be assigned the Part B and/or Part D penalty by the Medicare system automatically when you enroll in a Medicare Advantage plan.

Medicare Advantage Annual Enrollment

When you are older than 65, enrolling in an MA or an MAPD plan is fairly straightforward. You can enter into an MA during the Annual Election Period (AEP). That occurs every year during the fourth quarter. In 2012, the AEP runs from October 15 through December 7, a period of seven weeks. You will be able to freely change your mind, as many times as you would like. You can change your mind an infinite number of times, *and the last plan that you elect will be the plan that is in effect on the following January 1.* Since there is no restriction to the number of times that you can change your mind, it may be reasonable to choose the first plan so that you don't forget, and then you can go and shop around for different plans to the extent that you find the one that is superior to your initial selection. You may have misgivings about this, but the practical reality is that the Medicare system does the cancelling for you.

There are many other situations when enrollment into an MA or MAPD, even when not initially becoming eligible for Medicare Part A and Medicare Part B. There is a very long list conditions that qualify for Special Election Periods. The end section of this chapter will briefly discuss these SEPs.

Medicare Advantage Disenrollment Period

Sounds great, right? You can disenroll without restrictions between January 1 and February 14, every year. Now, here are the catches. First, if you have a PFFS plan, then you must request disenrollment. Second, you have to independently enroll in a stand-alone prescription drug plan (Medicare Part D). Fortunately, you are allowed to enroll in a stand-alone prescription drug plan (Medicare Part D) if you cancel during the disenrollment period.

Medicare Advantage 12-Month Trial Period

If you enroll in a Medicare Advantage plan during your open enrollment period, then you can cancel at any time during your first twelve months under that plan, and return to original Medicare. You can then enroll in a Medigap plan, or simply stay with original Medicare.

In addition, if the Medicare Initial Enrollment Period has expired, and you had cancelled your Medicare Advantage plan before your 12-month trial period ends, then you are able to select a PDP as well, which will be good until the following Annual Election Period (October 15-December 7). At that point, you can change your stand-alone PDP without restriction. If you cancel your MA during the 12-Month trial period, then you can select a new Medicare Part D plan, to be effective the 1st of the following month.

Note: Sometimes even insurance companies mishandle this situation, and do not process this as a Special Election Period under the twelve-month trial period.

Special Election Periods (SEP)

The Medicare system allows people that have special situations to be able to elect a Medicare Advantage plan outside the Annual Election Period.

Here is a list of 12 of them.

Moving: If you have moved, and your previous plan isn't offered in your new location, OR if you have moved and the new plan wasn't available in your old location, then you qualify. If you move from outside the U.S., where you were living permanently, then you qualify.

Medicaid Status Change: If your Medicaid status changes, then you qualify.

Limited Income Subsidy ("Extra Help"): If you are eligible for the Limited Income Subsidy, then you can change without restriction at any time during the calendar year.

Skilled Nursing Care Facility: If you are moving in OR out of a skilled nursing care facility, then you qualify.

PACE (Program of All-Inclusive Care for the Elderly): If you leave a PACE program, then you qualify. Note: PACE is only available in selected states.

Loss of Creditable Coverage: If your prescription drug benefits are ruled to no longer be creditable coverage, then you qualify. Note: "creditable coverage" is defined in the Glossary.

Employer-sponsored Plan Change: If you are losing your coverage from an employer-sponsored benefit plan, then you qualify. IMPORTANT NOTE: This is true whether or not it is voluntarily or involuntarily. You can choose to leave your plan and still qualify for this SEP. Do not accept any answer from any party, including the Social Security Administration, that informs you otherwise.

Pharmacy assistance program: If you are either entering a Qualified State Pharmaceutical Assistance Program (SPAP), or if you have lost your eligibility, then you qualify.

Other prescription drug assistance: If you no longer qualify for other prescription drug assistance that you have been receiving, then you qualify for an SEP.

Medicare Advantage Plan Cancellation: If your MA plan is no longer in existence, then you qualify (you must elect this SEP only between December 8 and the end of February of the following year).

Medicare Annual Disenrollment: Between January 1 and February 14, you can cancel, and return to original Medicare and enroll in a stand-alone prescription drug plan (Medicare Part D). If you have a PFFS, then you must obtain written permission.

Five Star Plan: If you want to switch to an MA plan that is rated as "five star" by the CMS, then you qualify, without calendar restriction. You can switch to a five star plan once, and only once, during a calendar year.

A general rule of thumb: If you qualify for an SEP, then you have 2 months from the date that you begin an SEP to adopt a new plan, whether that is another Medicare Advantage plan, or a new Medicare Part D plan, regardless of the reasons listed here.

Premiums

Medicare Advantage plans may have a monthly premium, which must be paid above and beyond the Medicare Part B monthly premium. Medicare Advantage plans will have a number of payment options, including taking a deduction directly from your Social Security payment, a coupon payment book, automatic bank deduction, a deduction from your Railroad Retirement Board check, as well as credit card.

If you rely on Medicaid or state assistance, it may be entirely possible that you can receive assistance to defray the costs of the Part B premium and the premium of an MA/MAPD. A person should check with their case worker to see if he/she is eligible for this assistance. Do not assume that you are ineligible, and do not assume that you will automatically be granted the assistance. It is beyond the scope of this book to fully examine SNPs. In some locations, there are Medicare Advantage plans which have zero (yes, $0) premium. This may be a very good alternative for a very select few.

Premiums have been relatively stable since the passage of the Patient Protection and Affordable Care Act (PPACA). However, the out-of-pocket costs, including deductibles and copays, i.e. cost sharing, has continued to weaken (i.e., worsen for the beneficiary, you). In 2013, this will weaken further, and in some cases, dramatically. Please read the Special Section at the end of this book for a further explanation. This is the difficulty with Medicare Advantage: ALL the terms and conditions are subject to change every year, and the premiums also change. When you add this to the terms of original Medicare worsening, it is difficult to measure the benefits of a particular Medicare Advantage against another. In some cases, certain Medicare Advantage plans are eliminated altogether for the following year. At that point, you have no other choice than to choose a new Medicare Advantage plan, or one will be chosen for you.

Deductibles and Coinsurance

Each Medicare Advantage plan will have its own cost sharing arrangements, a plan-specific set of terms and conditions. Those terms and conditions can require a certain schedule of payments for office visits (other than the preventative care checkup, which is complimentary under the Patient Protection and Affordable Care Act), hospital stays, skilled nursing care facilities, durable medical equipment, and everything else under Medicare Part A and Part B. Please know that the schedules must be fully detailed in your Summary of Benefits guide, and that the coverage that you receive in an MA or MAPD must be at least as good as the benefits that you receive under original Medicare. Lastly, there will be an annual out-of-pocket maximum amount. That annual out-of-pocket amount does not include amounts charged above the Medicare "allowed charge." The Medicare "allowed charge" has been described in Chapter 3.

All Medicare Advantage plans have received official approval from the CMS (Centers for Medicare & Medicaid Services). The cost sharing terms and conditions have been approved by the Centers for Medicare & Medicaid Services (CMS). Those amounts will limit your out-of-pocket expenses to a certain degree. Please note: the annual out-of-pocket maximum does not include the Part B Excess. There are no cases I have found in which a Medicare Advantage plan pays for an amount that exceeds the Medicare allowed charge.

In-Network vs. Out-of-Network

The most important aspect of Medicare Advantage (MA) coverage is the concept of network. Most people have experienced a network of some sort, whether that is in the form of your employer's group health insurance plan, or private health insurance. For MA, a similar concept applies. When you receive services from providers inside the network, cost sharing is reasonable. Outside the network, however, cost sharing greatly increases the out-of-pocket deductibles, copays, and annual out-of-pocket maximums. That is why it is important to check the physicians that you visit, as well as those that you might be reasonably expected to visit.

Doctors may or may not accept a particular Medicare Advantage plan; do not presume that your doctor will accept your Medicare

Advantage plan, even if he/she accepted your employer's plan in the past, and even if he/she accepted insurance from the same carrier before you were under Medicare. It is entirely separate, and you need to check this for yourself (or with an agent's assistance). HMOs, in particular, deserve very specific examination, because you can only go to a specialist upon your primary care provider's (PCP) recommendation. A useful analogy would be that in the past you drove a Lincoln, and now you drive a Ford. Well, it is the same in some ways (same manufacturer), but there will be many things that are entirely new. A similar thought should be applied here.

One thing that you must keep in mind is that if you travel on vacation, and you require medical attention, then that provider may or may not be inside the network.

This happens.

A "snowbird" (a person that goes to warm weather locations during the winter) may vacation for extended periods of time. However, when that person goes to his/her physician in Arizona (or Florida, etc), the physician may not belong to your network, and your out-of-network cost sharing arrangement would apply. That will be far more expensive than in-network, and the price differential can be so great, that it would have justified more comprehensive coverage via another selection.

This happens.

Not all insurance companies are equal, of course. Some are far more dominant in particular states, or in your particular location. Others are more national in scope and scale. You should think carefully if you're going to choose a Medicare Advantage plan, and check your medical providers *in advance* in order to minimize your out-of-pocket costs. Most of the time, the insurance companies have online directories, so you can search for your providers, or you can ask your insurance representative/agent for assistance.

In addition to that, you will be faced with a very complicated situation with respect to annual out-of-pocket maximums if you are enrolled in a Medicare Advantages. The reason this occurs is because some of your expenses will be in-network, and some will be out-of-network. You will need to be keep track of your visits, and the charges, and reconcile your statement of benefits that you receive from the insurance company that issued your Medicare Advantage plan. That alone is the source of great confusion because then you will basically be forced to verify your Medicare Advantage's records by comparing them to bills received.

Blue Cross Blue Shield

Perhaps the most widely known insurance company is Blue Cross Blue shield. Even though Blue Cross Blue Shield is a nationally-recognized label, the fact is that if you have a Medicare Advantage plan using Blue Cross Blue Shield, it is a state-by-state plan. In other words, a medical provider who accepts a Blue Cross plan in Florida may not be part of the Blue Cross plan in Illinois. Result? Do not presume that the medical provider who you go to in Florida is going to accept your Medicare Advantage plan if you were to travel out-of-state. You may incur out-of-network charges according to your Medicare Advantage's cost sharing plan.

What to Look For When Choosing Medicare Advantage

After reading *Maximize Your Medicare*, let's say that you have chosen a Medicare Advantage plan. Here are some important differences that exist among plans, and if correctly understood, you can either minimize your costs, or receive superior benefits.

Hospital stay deductible. There are two ways that most MA offer cost sharing if you are admitted to the hospital. You should choose the deductible that is a given cost per stay, and not the deductible that charges per day. Why is that? Simply put, you usually get admitted to a hospital for longer than a simple overnight stay. So when you multiply the per day copay times the number of days, that is usually more than the copay that is charged by those plans that charge on a per stay basis. All else equal, the premium will, on average, be slightly higher, but the fact is that if you stay at a hospital for multiple days, then you will save money by choosing an MA plan that charges you per stay.

Office visits. If there is a plan that does not distinguish between your family physician and a specialist, then that should be chosen, since an office visit to a specialist may be substantially more expensive than an office visit to your family doctor. In addition, remember that your annual examination is free, as a result of the Patient Protection and Affordable Care Act (PPACA).

Extra benefits. Many MA plans include discounts on dental and vision, weight-loss, and smoking cessation programs. Please know that extensive, specialized dental work, such as implants, or treatment of gum disease, are generally not covered by these extra benefits. In fact, as many of you know, serious dental work is usually uncovered by any type of dental insurance, or the maximum benefit is limited.

Five-Star Plans. The CMS rates plans every year. It is beyond the scope of this book to discuss how it reaches its determination. The plans are given a number of stars between 1 and 5. You can switch into a plan that has been given five stars by the CMS at any time during the year. This is a new Special Enrollment Period (SEP). You can switch into a five star program once, and only once, during a calendar year.

Last point: If you are a current enrollee in a Medicare Advantage plan, then you will receive a new copy of both an Annual Notice of Change (ANOC) and an Evidence of Coverage (EOC) guidebook. They will detail the changes for that Medicare Advantage plan for the next year, and compare it to the previous year's benefits. You should pay particular attention to the section that highlights the comparison of benefits from the current year to the next. If your benefits weaken, i.e. your cost sharing increases, then changing Medicare Advantage plans may be a good idea. It is not a good idea to simply file the notices away in a file cabinet, and find out that your out-of-pocket expenses have changed dramatically. By then, it is usually too late to make a change.

This is the fundamental problem with Medicare Advantage plans. We all know and accept that inflation occurs, and that healthcare costs are rising faster than inflation. There is no silver bullet for that problem. MA plans have two moving parts: prices and coverage. You cannot control Medicare's terms and condition of cost sharing (Part B deductible, Part A coinsurance and copays). What you have left is that you are left in the dark, every year, about the terms and conditions of both premiums and coverage. On the other hand, there is real competition in the marketplace. If anything, the Patient Protection and Affordable Care Act is proving to be a watershed for insurance companies, which will inevitably view Medicare Advantage and Medicare Supplemental insurance as a more stable, predictable business in which to be involved. Will that be enough to keep costs down? That, my friends, is an open question and unfortunately, Medicare Advantage enrollees learn a new answer every year.

Money Saving Tip #1 Medicare Advantage (You Get What You Pay For?)

There is the age-old saying, "You get what you pay for." Well, when it comes to Medicare Advantage, there is a new twist, and it goes, "You don't always get what you pay for, but you always pay for what you get." What in the world does this mean? It means that if you compare carefully, side-by-side (apples to apples, whatever), then you can find, even within the same company, that you can save premium, without a substantial decline in benefits. Maybe you have the time to compare by yourself, or maybe you know an expert, or a professional.

If you read the previous section, then you will find that you can obtain policies with similar out-of-pocket expenses and save $30-$50 a month. Maybe you think that isn't very much money. Now start multiplying by years and you will see the figures increase, and quickly. Anecdotally, people don't like change. They stay with the same plan if things do not change dramatically within their own plan. However, you need to remember that *there is intense competition among insurance companies*. You should absolutely use that to your advantage (no pun intended). Academic studies have concluded that consumers leave 10% a year in cost on prescription drug plans due to this behavior (lack of changing to more efficient plans). My thought is that this also occurs when it comes to Medicare Advantage plan selection. Take 10% a year, and start multiplying by years that you will live, and you will get the picture.

Of course, there are limits to this point, i.e. it is not the recommendation of *Maximize Your Medicare* that you change physicians every year in order to accommodate your Medicare Advantage plan. Nevertheless, not shopping around will cost you money, or benefits. If you need someone to do this for you, then find a professional. An agent worth his salt will be able to easily figure it out.

Chapter 5. Medicare Part D (Prescription Drug Plans)

Stand-alone prescription drug plans (PDPs) are also known as Medicare Part D. Sometimes, the terminology can be complicated. For those enrolled in an MAPD, a separate Part D plan is unnecessary. In fact, the Medicare system will not allow you to have multiple prescription plans.

Enrollment

For those that are newly eligible for Medicare Part A and Part B, the Medicare Initial Enrollment Period applies. In our "Jane Doe" case, she turns 65 on February 13, 2013. That means she can enroll in Part D plans as early as November 1, 2012, and as late as May 31, 2013, without incurring a penalty.

After May 31, 2013, "Jane Doe" will begin to incur a penalty if she has not enrolled in Medicare Part D. The Medicare Part D penalty rate is 1% for every month that you do not enroll. The amount of the penalty is based on the national average of the price of a prescription drug plan, not on the 1% of the plan that you select. Additionally, *the penalty never expires.* Let's start with an example. Say you choose an inexpensive prescription drug plan. The penalty will not be based on your plan's premium. So if the average drug plan costs $30 then your 1% would be $.30 for every month that you did not enroll in the plan during your open enrollment.

You can have Medicare Part A and Part D only, if you so choose.

Premiums

Premiums are indexed to income, which means that if you earn more than $85,000 as an individual, or greater than $170,000 filing jointly, you can be charged more for your Part D. The additional amount is called the Income-Related Monthly Adjustment Amount (IRMAA). The IRMAA will automatically be deducted from your Social Security benefit. Complete details on the amount are found in Table 3 at the end of this chapter.

Here are the terms of Medicare Part D:

$0-$325: If the costs are between $0 and $325 in a calendar year, then the Medicare Part D is paid according to the plan that you purchase. Premiums, deductibles, and copays vary by plan. Applicants should check on the website www.medicare.gov in order to find out which Medicare Part D plans cover the drugs that the applicant takes.

$325-$2930: You pay a co-pay of the total costs of prescriptions between $325 and $2930. The Medicare Part D provider and you combine to pay the reminder, depending upon the Medicare Part D you select.

$2930-$4700: In 2013, there is a 52% discount on covered brand-name prescription drugs. You will pay a maximum of 86% for the cost of generic drugs while in this gap. This is called the Coverage Gap by CMS, and is commonly referred to as the "donut hole." The important thing here is that certain stand-alone prescription plans provide for partial coverage inside the donut hole. If this is you, and you know in advance that you will fall within the donut hole, then it is most likely the case that you should choose a plan with a higher premium, which will result in lower overall costs throughout a calendar year.

$4700+: You pay 5% of the total costs of prescriptions above $4700. The Medicare Part D provider pays the remainder. This is called catastrophic coverage.

Choosing the Right Plan

Once you have decided to enroll in the prescription drug plan then the question is what is the best plan for you. This is will require some work on your part. You may request the assistance of an agent. You can do it yourself by going to https://medicare.gov/find-a-plan/questions/home.aspx. Here are the steps to take.

1. Enter your zip code.
2. Choose the "I don't know what coverage I have" selection, and choose the "I don't know" selection. Click on the "Continue to Plan Results."
3. You will be sent to Step 2 of 4: Enter Your Drugs page. Follow directions. Enter the drugs and the dosages that you require. Once completed, click "My Drug List is Complete."
4. You will be sent to Step 3 of 4: Select Your Pharmacies. Choose pharmacies from the list. When complete, click "Continue to Plan Results."
5. There will be three categories. The one to choose is the FIRST ONE, called "Prescription Drug Plans (with original Medicare)."
6. The results will come out under "Prescription Drug Plans."

The results will be in order; the least expensive plans are listed first. The results are estimates only. Helpful hint: You do not need to do this more than once. Write down the Drug List ID and Password Date listed near the top of the website. It can be used again to recall the list of prescriptions that you have input into the site.

Here are some general concepts to understand regarding stand-along prescription drug plans (PDPs). Some prescription drug plans will require the beneficiary to pay the annual deductible. Some will not. Your medication may or may not be covered. That will result in higher out-of-pocket costs, but every plan must cover at least two medications per medical condition. (If your drug is not covered by your plan, there can be exceptions. This can occur when your doctor writes a letter to essentially appeal your case.)

Different copayments will exist for each drug, and it will not be the same across plans. That is why you need the assistance of the Medicare.gov website or an insurance agent. Paper copies of the formularies that itemize the medications covered by your MAPD plans are sent before the Annual Election Period to enrollees.

For those with very extensive medications that are new to the market, the formularies (list of approved medications) can change within a calendar year. If you are directed by your physician to take one of these, then you should call your Part D provider to ask. In addition, those with expensive medications need to work with insurance companies because the insurance companies may expect you to participate in a therapy program to make sure that you are not taking an unnecessarily-expensive medication for an extended period.

If you do not have access to the internet, then you can ask an insurance agent or broker to do this for you. If he/she can't or won't, then here is a piece of advice: find another agent who will.

Preferred Pharmacies and Mail Order

Prescription plans often use preferred pharmacies, and should be used whenever possible. When you select a stand-alone prescription drug plan, it is important to input those pharmacies that you frequently use. Then, and only then, will you receive an accurate list of the cheapest plans. The same can be said for mail order. Most Part D plans have a mail order option for many prescriptions, and these can reduce out-of-pocket expenses dramatically. That said, some people are not comfortable in receiving prescriptions via mail. Certain medications have a very high "street value," especially in the case of pain management medications, and special care must be taken in delivery of these sensitive drugs.

Changing Plans

You can change your Part D plan during every Annual Election Period (AEP) without restriction. That means that if your prescriptions change during the year, the best plan may also change. This is important to keep in mind. Even if your prescriptions do not change throughout the year, you should still check to confirm that your plan is the best for you. The reason? Premiums will change, copays will change, drug coverage will change for different plans on an annual basis. This means that the plan that fits you best may also change. It may be costly to not check (see the "Money-Saving Tip").

The Coverage Gap ("Donut Hole") and You

The Coverage Gap is commonly referred to as the "Donut Hole." It is described above in the description of Part D plans. Frankly, it receives more attention than it deserves, because the vast majority of people will take generic medications whenever possible, and the result is that the donut hole will not be a factor. However, "donut hole" is a snappy piece of jargon which is useful at the coffee shop amongst friends. That all said, here are the situations that describe the vast majority of Medicare-eligible.

The donut hole is irrelevant if your prescription costs, including premium are less than $2930 during the calendar year. You will follow your Part D plan. Be sure to read the Money-Saving tips at the end of this chapter.

However, when you have paid a total of $2930, then you enter the donut hole. For 2013, your prescription drug plan converts to a fixed schedule where you have to pay 47.5% at most for non-generic drugs, 14% of the cost for generic drugs. You will receive a 52.5% discount for non-generic medications. This continues until the total costs reach $4700. Once you have reached $4700, catastrophic coverage begins, and the price is 5% of the cost for non-generic medications. That is obviously a great deal of money, and it starts all over again every calendar year. Certain plans have partial coverage gap protection. It should not be surprising that those with partial coverage gap benefits usually are accompanied by higher monthly premiums than those plans without coverage gap benefits. The important thing is to not simply choose a plan based on its lower premium; that may result in higher prescription costs over an entire year due to higher copays.

The controversy around the donut hole is not likely to recede anytime soon. It is the subject of considerable debate in Washington D.C. For those that receive prescription coverage from other sources, it may be reason to stay with a group plan or retiree group coverage. Please see the next section called "Employer Group Plans and the Coverage Gap ('Donut Hole')," where this complicated matter is addressed.

Employer Group Plans and the Coverage Gap ("Donut Hole")

Please note: an entire chapter is devoted to employer-sponsored group plans for Medicare-eligible employees and retirees. Nothing here is inconsistent with that section, and if you have an employer-sponsored group plan, then you should refer to that chapter.

The important question about the donut hole is how it may be better or worse than your existing prescription plan. In certain employer plans, there is no concept of donut hole. That means that if your drug costs are very high and you compare your estimate of annual costs under Medicare Part D to how much you would pay through your employer plan, the drug portion may be cheaper in your employer plan than it would be under a stand-alone Part D (prescription drug plan).

As a result, the fact is that you may want to stay with your employer plan. However, it isn't always that simple. Sometimes persons come to me and tell me, "I want to stay with my employer due to the fact that the drug cost will be lower." This may be true, OR NOT. *At the risk of being repetitive, I repeat: do not assume that the best case is staying with your employer-provided plan.* It is financial reality that you, as a retiree, are not the priority. If you conclude that this is the case, after asking the right questions, then it is fine for you to stay with your retiree plan. Not before examining the facts. I will show you why this is the case.

There are employer-provided plans that still have a donut hole that is *identical* to the Medicare "donut hole." Even if there is no donut hole, it may not be entirely clear that this is reason enough to stay with an employer group plan. Your prescription savings need to be compared to the savings that you might have gotten on superior medical plans in the private market as a whole. Remember: medical coverage in the private market is frequently superior to the coverage in a group plan. Therefore, your employer-provided medical benefits must be weighed against the medical plan that you would have under an MA or a Medigap plan. On balance, the medical coverage and cost sharing arrangement under an MAPD or Medigap plan may be worth the extra cost under the prescription plan. That has to be done on a case-by-case basis and there is no shortcut to it.

An advisor or an agent may be useful in this case because he/she would be able to add up the plan's costs, as well as their benefits, for you, so that you choose the best overall plan. **It is vital that Medicare-eligible persons understand that the two components (medical and prescription) be considered in combination, and not one without regard to the other.**

The reason that is important to consider both the prescription plan as well as your medical plan together is that if you are concerned about the high cost of prescriptions, then it is usually the case that you have a medical situation which requires constant attention. One common mistake is that people ignore the *correlation between prescription costs and the medical services they require.* The reason that people get rejected by private insurance companies before becoming Medicare-eligible is that insurance companies do not make this mistake. Insurance companies know that, given a list of medications, it may suggest that further medical services will be required in the future.

The savings that you will receive as a result of superior medical coverage using a Medigap plan may be greater than the savings under a prescription plan or the drug plan included as part of an employer-sponsored plan. So fine, you save a few hundred dollars on prescriptions, but the risk is that you have thousands of extra dollars of medical bills. The very person that requires more medications is the same person that is more likely to incur medical bills.

Extra Help Program

"Extra Help" is a program sponsored by the federal government. If you qualify, then the Extra Help program can pay a portion of your Medicare prescription drug costs. The Extra Help program may pay all or part of your monthly Medicare Part D plan premiums and a significant portion of your medication costs.

In addition, you will also pay either a low or no initial deductible and will not be subject to the Coverage Gap ("donut hole") of Medicare Part D as described in Chapter 5. You do not have the same restriction as others if you qualify for the Extra Help program, i.e. you can change plans at any time during the year, without restriction. Put another way, if you are in the Extra Help program, then your entire year is an SEP.

If you qualify for the Extra Help program, then you need to be aware that there a number of different levels of assistance. It is beyond the scope of this book to detail the income and net worth requirements for each level. You will be (or should have been) audited by a case worker once a year. In addition, you need to check the letters (don't discard them!) that you receive in order to understand your individual level of assistance, which is subject to change, every year.

Every year, you may receive a letter from Social Security Administration, which will update you on your status. You may be told that you do not qualify for the next year. If this is the case, then this is one type of Special Election Period (SEP), and you will be able to adjust your selection of Part D, as well as enroll in an MA plan, or a Medigap plan. You may receive a letter requesting additional information; **this is a very important letter (which is one reason to never throw away letters from the CMS), because if you do not answer the letter, then you can lose your access to the Extra Help program entirely.**

Money-Saving Tip #1 and 2013 Update

Many people choose a stand-alone prescription drug plan (Medicare Part D), and then, simply due to convenience, a Medicare beneficiary simply chooses to stay with the same plan. Given the other advice contained in this book, you can anticipate my reaction to this: *bad idea.* It would be better to check your annual costs using the steps listed in "Choosing the Right Plan" every year. The reason is that *not changing costs you*, on average, 10% a year on your premiums. That is the conclusion of the study conducted by Keith M. Marzilli Ericson in a working paper, published in September 2012, of the National Bureau of Economic Research (NBER), the nation's foremost collection of economists. Bottom line: check your list of prescriptions annually, and use the directions as listed in "Choosing the Right Plan" every year.

Even in cases when your prescriptions stay the same, the cost sharing arrangement can change for the same plan. In 2013, premiums are higher, and perhaps more significantly, the copays are worse than in 2012. For example, instead of a percentage there may be a copay schedule; some very large, popular Part D plans are changing to a fixed dollar amount. That is a problem because if you have a non-generic medication that costs $80/month, and during 2012, you had to pay 25%, or $20 a month, this year your plan may have a fixed copay for that medication that is $60 a month, in which case you would be paying $40 extra, a month, for that one prescription. In certain cases, that will be up to an additional $480 per year that you will need to pay from your personal funds. The headlines that you can read regarding Part D, then, do not tell the whole story.

Money-Saving Tip #2: Shingles Vaccination and Part D

Shingles, as many know, is very closely related to the well-known childhood illness chickenpox. The science isn't that important. What is important: left undetected, shingles has exceptionally painful side effects. At extremes, morphine is prescribed for pain management purposes. It is that bad. Fortunately, a vaccine exists. Unfortunately, the cost is quite high. You should check your local pharmacy.

Why is this related to Medicare Part D? This vaccination is largely covered under Medicare Part D, but the cost sharing of this expensive vaccination varies. All else equal, you can choose a plan without annual deductible, and as a result, the copay on the shingles vaccination will be lower than under plans where you must pay the $325 annual deductible.

The difference can easily be $150 savings for the one shot alone. That equates to $12.50 a month (=$150 / 12). When you compare premiums, this type of out-of-pocket expense needs to be taken into consideration. For a person that takes no medications, the lowest priced plans are approximately $10/month lower than the lowest-priced plan without a deductible.

For people that take the most common generics, the total costs may be the same, assuming that your prescriptions do not change throughout the year. However, what happens if you are prescribed a more expensive medication? *Then, on average, the higher priced plan, with no deductible, will result in lower overall costs because the copay structure of higher-premium plans is usually superior. You will need to confirm that (and all other facts stated in this book), but it illustrates the point that the lowest monthly premium plan may not be as obvious as it seems.*

Table 3. Medicare Part D Cost Sharing (2013)

Individual	Joint	Monthly Premium
$85,000 or less	$170,000 or less	Plan Premium
$85,001 - $107,000	$170,001 - $214,000	$11.60 + Plan Premium
$107,001 - $160,000	$214,001 - $320,000	$29.90 + Plan Premium
$160,001 - $214,000	$320,000 - $428,000	$48.10 + Plan Premium
Greater than $214,000	Greater than $428,000	$66.40 + Plan Premium

Additional amounts ($11.60, $29.90, $48.10, $66.40) will automatically deducted from your Social Security benefits (if applicable).

Source: CMS

Chapter 6. Medigap, Medicare Supplemental

Now we proceed to looking at Medigap, otherwise known as Medicare Supplements, or Medicare Supplemental insurance. Those are three different terms but they are all the same thing; they all describe the same set of plans I will discuss with you. You will need to be enrolled in both Medicare Part A and Part B. This chapter will describe the general terms and conditions of those plans, as well as the enrollment timeline. I will also discuss what is covered and not covered. Ultimately I will describe to you the advantages that Medigap plans offer, as well as some highlights of individual Medigap plans. The conclusion will be that Medigap plans, along with a stand-alone prescription drug plan (PDP) may be better for you than any other configuration that exists in the market today.

During Medicare Open Enrollment

Medigap Open Enrollment

The Medigap open enrollment period is not the same as the Medicare Initial Enrollment Period. The Medigap open enrollment period begins on the first day of the month that you become eligible for Medicare Part B, and it lasts for six months. For Medicare Advantage as well as Medicare Part D (stand-alone prescription drug plan), this is a very important fact to keep in mind.

Remember Jane Doe, born on February 13, 1948? She turns 65 years old on February 13, 2013. The way that Medigap open enrollment period works is her open enrollment period begins on February 1, 2013 and it lasts through July 31, 2013.

This may seem strange, since the Medicare Advantage (Medicare Part C) open enrollment period begins on November 1, 2012. Depending on the state, you can apply prior to the beginning of the Medigap open enrollment period. Huh? February 1, 2012 is the beginning of Jane Doe's Medigap open enrollment period. She can apply in advance. That will depend on the state and/or insurance company. Easy rule of thumb: when the Medicare Initial Coverage Election Period (ICEP) begins, you can usually sign up for Medigap (see "Money Savings Tips on Medigap" below). Money-saving tip: in certain cases, you can sign up for Medigap even before you can apply for Medicare Advantage, and you may be able to save additional money by doing so. This is entirely up to the individual insurance company, but the practical reality is that many companies allow you to enroll well before you enter the official Medigap open enrollment period.

In theory, you could have Medicare Part A and Part B only and then you could wait for five more months and then you could enter into Medigap with no penalty. It is not my opinion that this is the path that should be taken, but it is an option. Please note: even if you deliberately wait until the end of the Medigap open enrollment period, that does not change the Medicare Part D open enrollment period. For our Jane Doe, the last day to enroll in Part D is May 31, 2012, regardless of the date that she applies for a Medigap policy.

Medigap Guaranteed Issue

During the Medigap open enrollment period, you are guaranteed to be issued the Medigap policy of your choice. You are entitled during this very special time; **IF YOU ARE SERIOUSLY ILL WITH A KNOWN CONDITION THAT YOU KNOW WILL REQUIRE CONSTANT CARE, USE THE OPEN ENROLLMENT PERIOD TO OBTAIN THE MOST COMPREHENSIVE PROTECTION THAT YOU CAN AFFORD.**

During the Medigap open enrollment period, insurance companies cannot deny you coverage, nor can they charge you a higher price based on your medical situation. While insurance companies are obligated to accept you, however, they can charge different prices based on gender, height, weight, and tobacco use. That is the current trend and until 2014 when the Patient Protection and Affordable Care Act (PPACA) is enacted, it is reasonable to anticipate that this will continue. You can observe this phenomenon now; insurers are charging different prices for different genders, smoking and non-smoking, and finally, they're asking you about your body mass index (BMI), in which case you look at a chart for your height and weight. Depending on your categories, you will be guaranteed coverage, but at a different prices. This does not mean that you will be denied. You will be entitled to buy, but at a higher price.

Enrolling in Medigap During Other Periods

Switching From One Medigap Policy to Another

This is possible. However, you will be subject to medical underwriting. An insurance company can choose to accept or deny coverage based on your answers to medical questions.

Switching From Medicare Advantage to Medigap

If it is during the Annual Election Period (AEP), this is possible, subject to medical underwriting. An insurance company can choose to accept or deny coverage based on your answers to medical questions. If your Medicare Advantage does not include prescription drug benefits, then you can switch, subject to medical underwriting, at any time during the year. If your Medicare Advantage does include prescription drug benefits, then you should wait for the Annual Election Period, because you will be cancelling your prescription drug benefits, and you cannot enroll in a stand-alone prescription drug plan (Medicare Part D) until the Annual Election Period (AEP).

How Medigap Works with Original Medicare

Medigap plans come with letters A-N. The different plans, what they cover, what they do not cover; it is in the chart at the end of this chapter. Every Medigap plan must at least cover what Medicare Part A covers. This section highlights the benefits you receive as a Medigap policyholder.

Medigap and Medicare Part A

You can see in Table 4 that every Medigap plan will pay, either in full or in part, the Part A deductibles. That makes every Medigap plan vastly better than original Medicare. You may remember from the Chapter 2 (on Medicare Part A), that the deductible for hospital admission is $1184 per benefit period. In all plans except Plan K, Plan L, and High-deductible Plan F, the entire deductible is paid. This compares very favorably with original Medicare and Medicare Advantage plans.

In addition, all Medigap plans will cover at least 50% of the copay amount from days 21 to 100 in a skilled nursing care facility. For example, if you have a joint replacement surgery, and you enter a rehabilitation center for a period longer than expected, then your Medigap plan will cover at least 50% of the $148 a day that the Medicare system does not under the current system.

The $148 per day copay for days 21-100 is reset annually, so the daily charge may be larger through time. Again, this is favorable when compared to Medicare Advantage, which may require a copayment on a daily basis.

My Opinion: It is likely that the cost sharing terms of admission to a skilled nursing care facility will worsen in 2013 when compared to 2012. This makes intuitive sense; it is very common for people to receive joint replacement surgery as they age, and that requires rehabilitation. More people requiring rehabilitation means higher prices. Period.

Medigap Medicare Part B

With respect to Medicare Part B, you can see again by Table 4 that many of the Medigap plans cover most, if not all, of what is not covered by the Medicare Part B. For example, the C and F plans cover the annual deductible, which is currently $147. Again, please note that if a plan covers the Medicare Part B deductible and the Part B deductible increases, then that plan will cover whatever the Part B deductible is for that year.

Coinsurance that accompanies Medicare Part B is paid in full by all Medigap plans except K and L, in which the Medigap pays 50% (or 75% for Plan L) of the 20% that original Medicare Part B does not pay. For all other plans (except for High-Deductible Plan F which is described later in this chapter), a Medigap policy pays for the entire 20% that is not covered by Medicare Part B.

One particular Medigap plan (Plan N) charges a fee per office visit. I refer to Table 4 again, and you can see it's a maximum of $20 for most office visits. To be clear, the annual preventative care examination is still free, in accordance with the Patient Protection and Affordable Care Act (PPACA). The $147 Medicare Part B deductible is for services received, but *not* the annual preventative care visit. The complimentary annual preventative care visit is governed by the Patient Protection and Affordable Care Act (PPACA). For emergency room visits, it is a $50 per visit to an emergency room, which is refunded to you if you are admitted to the hospital, because then you would fall under Part A.

A Few Exceptions

You will notice that not all letters are represented, because some plans have been discontinued by the Medicare system. All plans are authorized by the CMS, the Centers for Medicare & Medicaid Services. The terms of coverage for the different plans are identical across all insurance companies whether that insurance company is Aetna, Transamerica, etc. Since they are all identical to each other, you can compare prices easily. Generally, this should be the source of great comfort to consumers. However, there are some twists to this, and they will be addressed at the end of this chapter. One extra twist that will be described at the end of the chapter is called the pre-existing condition waiting period.

There are a few exceptions to the way that Medigap policies work in certain states. In some states, you may be able to buy another type of Medigap policy called Medicare SELECT. SELECT plans are standardized plans that may require you to see certain providers and may cost less than other plans. You can be charged more if you receive services that are not part of a pre-specified list.

Attained-Age vs Issue-Age vs Community-Age

There are three different pricing mechanisms for Medigap policies. They are attained-age, issue-age and community-age. In reality, they are quite straightforward to understand. The availability of the different types of plans varies depending on your state. This book will address the three types in order of popularity.

Attained-age has a separate price depending upon your actual age. Let's revisit Jane Doe, who becomes eligible on February 1, 2013. She will be offered a price for a 65-year-old woman. Depending upon the insurance company, the premium may stay constant for a pre-stated period of time. Insurance companies have the right to change premiums as long as they can prove that claims are 80% of the premiums minus administrative and other various charges. The important fact is that when Jane turns 66 years old, she can be charged a different premium. She cannot be charged a different premium based on her individual claims.

Community-age has a single price regardless of age. It does not differ whether you are 65 years old or 80 years old. This has an obvious advantage, which is that as you get older, it may make sense to have a community-age based Medigap policy, if you are allowed to do so. That said, the premium of a community-age policy should be expectedly higher than the attained-age policy for the same person who is new to Medicare. The other issue to consider is that even though the price is not different if you are 65 or 80 years old, the price for the entire community of policyholders may increase as a whole.

Issue-age policies are priced when you first purchase the plan, and the price does not change. Like community-age policies, issue-age policies have a price that is initially higher than the more popular attained-age.

It is almost impossible to predict which type of pricing will work out best over the long run. On one hand, lower premiums are undoubtedly better, all else being equal. That would imply that attained-age is best. In addition, you may think, "Well, if I don't live that long, then I don't have to worry about the much higher premiums at much later ages." This line of reasoning is intuitively attractive, to be sure.

On the other hand, if there are structural changes to Medicare, such as dramatic changes to the coinsurance and copays (cost sharing), then premiums that don't increase may be the superior solution. In addition, there are certain locations where a particular insurance company issuing a community-age Medigap policy cannot raise rates for a specified period of time. In certain states, the price of a community-age based plan is fixed for a certain period of time. That, of course, is the best of all worlds, especially if the Medigap plan is the one that you prefer.

Base Case: Medigap is Superior to Medicare Advantage

If you read the introduction to this book you can remember that my main objective here for you is for you to avoid catastrophic losses. Some events, like a hurricane, cannot be anticipated. Of course, no one wants to get ill. However, if it occurs, as is more likely as you naturally age, then catastrophic losses can add up, and cost you a significant portion of your retirement savings. No one can avoid the natural aging process, and the increased likelihood of getting ill that accompanies the passage of time. I'm trying to have you avoid the substantially higher costs that could occur if you get ill, so that you can enjoy your retirement years.

If you can afford it, then Medigap and a stand-alone prescription drug plan is best, particularly when you first become Medicare-eligible. Even a Medigap Plan N is superior to most MAPD plans, for very similar prices. At the end of the day, Medigap plans do a superior job of covering Medicare Part A costs under original Medicare. If you enter into a situation when the Part A deductible or coinsurance are due, then Medigap will end up saving you money, and there is no concept of network, the point mentioned earlier. For those of you that don't like the guesswork of calculating how much you will owe when you receive medical services from your physician, Medigap provides clarity and consistency. The benefits provided by your Medigap policy next year will be calculated the same way it is calculated this year.

Advantages of Medigap

Why would I recommend so strongly for persons to enter into a Medigap policy as soon as they are able to do so? The answer is that once you are out of your Medigap open enrollment period, individual insurance companies are able to ask you questions regarding your health, and deny you coverage if you wanted to purchase a Medigap plan. There may be some selected companies that will accept you, even if you have pre-existing conditions. **Those are the insurance companies that you will want to avoid, if you can, due to the way in which insurance companies establish their premiums.**

If you have Type 1 diabetes, for example, most insurance companies will not offer you Plan F after the Medigap open enrollment period ends. Those that do are well-known to have premiums that rise dramatically faster than its competitors in the marketplace. It remains to be seen how this will change upon enactment of the Patient Protection and Affordable Care Act.

Even under a Special Election Period (SEP), individual insurance companies may be allowed to deny coverage under certain plans, as long as they offer Plan A, and one of Plan C or Plan F. If you disenroll from a group plan for any reason, you will have the right (for up to two months after that plan is cancelled/discontinued) to enter into a Medigap policy under a Special Election Period. In addition to the ability to purchase a Medigap policy, the SEP will allow you to enter into a stand-alone prescription drug plan (PDP/ Medicare Part D).

This happens.

A 67-year-old is informed that his retiree health insurance plan is going to be cancelled by his employer. He wants to choose a Medigap policy. He faces two issues. First, he may be asked medical qualifying questions depending on the individual insurance company and the Medigap policy he would like. That means his choices may be more limited than if he had enrolled into a Medigap policy during the Medigap open enrollment period.

There is another reason. Even if he were in perfect health at 67-years-old, the plan that he originally wanted may not even exist at the time that he wants to change into Medigap. Remember that the design of Medigap policies is governed by the Centers for Medicare & Medicaid Services (CMS). That means that CMS also has the right to discontinue plans; it has done this in the past. Plans D, E - a prime example is E - H, I, and J Plans no longer exist (although original policy owners still can use their plans as long as they continue to pay premiums).

This happens.

No Network, No Annual Election Period

Unlike Medicare Advantage plans, Medigap has no concept of network at all. If your medical doctor or medical provider accepts Medicare, then they're required by law to accept Medigap. Sometimes, you will get pushback from a secretary, who asks you what Medigap plan you may have. This is actually quite annoying for a billing professional to ask, because that actually isn't a relevant question. It isn't even a question that they should be asking you. I repeat: if a doctor or medical provider accepts Medicare assignment, they are required *by law* to accept your Medigap policy, regardless of location.

One other additional point is that many of the plans under Medigap actually allow for foreign travel emergency services. There is a $250 deductible. Your Medigap policy will pay for 80% of your emergency travel medical expenses, up to a lifetime maximum $50,000. You are responsible for the remainder of the bill. Candidly, *you will probably need to wait to be reimbursed.* It may be cumbersome, from a practical point of view, to file a claim while you are in a foreign country, so you will be able to file claims with your insurance company after you return home.

Medigap and the Part B Excess Charge

Earlier, the Medicare Part B Excess Charges were explained. Recall that a medical provider can charge up to 15% more than the Medicare-allowed charge, and the out-of-pocket costs can be very high. Under Medigap Plans F, High-Deductible F, and G, the Medicare Part B Excess Charges are covered in full. If you have Plan F or plan G, and the doctor charges more than the Medicare "allowed charge," then your Medigap will cover this amount. For high-deductible Plan F, the Part B excess charge is paid after you meet the annual deductible, which is $2,070 in 2012.

We need to examine this particular piece of information, because generally speaking F and G are more expensive than the other plans. Now, the question is, is the protection provided worth the cost? On one hand, these plans can be $400-800 more per year in premium than other Medigap plans. There is no doubt that this is a lot of money. However, if you are a person with an incurable disease, such as Parkinson's disease, diabetes (Type 1), cancer, Rheumatoid Arthritis, Congestive Heart Failure, or Multiple Sclerosis, then you are facing a fairly long period in which you will require extensive medical attention. If you suffer a heart attack requiring open heart surgery, or if you suffer a stroke, then again, there will be a long, difficult to recovery. If one episode occurs like this in your lifetime, the $400-800 dollars a year can be paid many times over, depending on the treatment required.

In addition to the financial considerations, there is also the emotional aspect that has not been mentioned in this book, as yet. Persons that face serious medical conditions require not only their own strength, but the strength their family and friends. It could easily be said that there is almost no price tag that can be put on peace of mind. There will not be an endless trail of medical bills, there will not be any worries about how to pay, and there will not be any thoughts about the financial costs on those around you.

Standardization and Grandfathering

The previous example highlights two important features of Medigap policies. I will call them standardization and grandfathering. By standardization, the coverage for all Plan N's is the same, regardless of insurance company. That also makes it easier for medical provider administrators/billing personnel to understand. The idea of language that changes from company to company or hidden language simply does not exist. The second and potentially more important reason that a Medigap policy is superior to any other policy is because of the grandfathering characteristic. As long as you continue to pay premiums then the policy remains in effect as it was originally conceived, unless it is changed by the CMS. Maybe you think that this is irrelevant. Think again.

In the past, the Medicare system has discontinued plans but has allowed persons who were originally enrolled in that plan to stay with the same language. That's very important, largely because of the fact that we may anticipate, or reasonably predict, that the Medicare system will change in the future. As you may have read, doomsday predictions suggest that the Medicare system will be insolvent as soon as 2016. For the record, I don't think this is a plausible scenario (the most influential voting bloc is over 50 years old). However, it is entirely possible, if not probable, that certain plans may be discontinued in the future. The point? There is no better time than now to lock down the coverage, which would take advantage of the grandfathering characteristic (mentioned in the previous section) that you will desire over the long run. If you wait for that period of time to arrive before changing, you may be rejected for medical reasons, or perhaps the plans that you desire may not exist at all.

When Is Medicare Advantage Better Than Medigap?

More comprehensive medical coverage and consistency of costs are the two largest reasons for choosing Medigap instead of Medicare Advantage. However, there are some situations in which MA may be the better option. As mentioned earlier, Medicare Advantage can offer additional benefits, such as discounts for smoking-cessation programs, weight-loss programs, and vision and dental discounts, among others. While in the short run, these may give you some satisfaction, you will quickly forget your discounted trips to the fitness center if you are admitted to the hospital and have large out-of-pocket expenses. You can compare the cost sharing of Medicare Advantage, to Medigap, and see for yourself.

You Are Financially Stretched

Maximize Your Medicare does not mean minimize your food. It is another way of saying that I am not advocating you becoming "insurance poor." You need to eat, pay bills, and live. There are other priorities in life as well. Perhaps you have to support someone else. Maybe you think it is more important to buy your grandchildren clothes. It isn't the role of *Maximize Your Medicare* to determine this for you. On the other hand, remember that you need to be in good health in order to contribute to others. That is for you to decide. With that in mind, there are reasons that Medicare Advantage could be a superior choice when compared to Medigap.

You can easily find Medicare Advantage plans that are cheaper than Medigap. MA is convenient, especially because prescription drug benefits are frequently combined with medical insurance. If you receive prescription drug benefits from another source, then the price of an MA plan without prescription coverage may make sense. In certain states, HMOs actually rebate you part of your Medicare Part B premium. This fact implies that the Medicare

Part B premium for 2013 will be higher than in 2012. While the Part B Excess has been explained, and the risks have also been explained, you may be willing to accept that risk and the inferior cost sharing arrangements of Medicare Advantage because you need to save the extra money. One objective of this book is to point out that Medigap policies can be found that are essentially the same price as Medicare Advantage plans, and that due to the consistency of coverage, along with unwritten implications, Medigap is superior to Medicare Advantage. All else equal, then, Medigap would be the better choice.

However, "all else equal" may be language that does not apply. At some price, it may be worth it to accept the inferior cost sharing terms within Medicare Advantage plans. It isn't the role of this book, or an agent, to make that judgment for you. Financial priorities may dictate your choices. This is economic reality; this book is written so that you know what the risks are of the choices that you make.

You Are Well Over 70 Years Old

The most popular, most widely available Medigap plans are attained-age, as described earlier in this chapter. Medicare Advantage plans are entirely community-age based. That means that premiums of Medicare Advantage do not change, regardless of age. They are reset every year, and it doesn't matter if you are 65 or 85, the price is the same.

It may be that the price differential between Medigap and MA, when you reach advanced ages, makes a change from Medigap to MA a very good idea. However, remember that the conditions stated in the previous section ("Base Case: Medigap is Superior to Medicare Advantage") are still true. The language will change and the premium will change every year, and the Part B excess remains uncovered. It is not easy, and depends very much on the amount of financial resources you have. If you cannot afford the premiums, and find that you are being stretched financially as a result of Medigap premiums as you reach an advanced age, then a change to an MA plan may a good idea.

You Always Stay Close to Home

As stated above, one drawback of Medicare Advantage is the idea that there is a network. Cost sharing is worse if you want to receive services from a provider that is not in your network. In extreme cases (as in an HMO), you would need to bear the entire costs not covered by original Medicare. In other cases, receiving services from an out-of-network provider can be double the cost when compared to receiving services from an in-network provider.

However, if you do not travel at all, and your providers are the same ones that you have used for a long time, and the facilities in your area are ones that will not change, then you may not use the advantages that a Medigap policy offers. In that case, perhaps the extra benefits that often accompany an MA plan are more worthwhile than the flexibility that you get due to absence of a network. That is entirely possible if you don't travel away from home.

Money-Saving Tips on Medigap

Enroll in Medigap Early

Let's start with a little review. A fact mentioned earlier in this chapter is that insurance companies will allow you to enroll in a Medigap policy well before your first date of Medicare eligibility. Do you remember Jane Doe? Her first date of Medicare eligibility is February 1, 2013. Her Medigap open enrollment period begins February 1, 1948, but insurance companies frequently allow clients to apply for Medigap well in advance of that. In addition, insurance companies may allow her to pay premiums well in advance.

If you have the ability to do so, then you can pay *before* the premium increase takes effect by enrolling early, by enrolling before price changes are announced.

Renew Your Medigap Early

Every year, Medigap premiums generally change on January 1 (and then again when you change attained age). Usually, those rates are established sometime during the end of the year. For example, you can expect insurance companies to post their rates for 2013 sometime during November through December. However, many insurance companies will allow you to pay your premiums in advance, for up to 12 months. If you have the resources available, then you can avoid a year's increase by paying your premium in advance, for as far as you can, and as far as your insurance company will allow.

High-Deductible Plan F May Be a Bargain

There are only 3 plans that will cover the Medicare Part B Excess. They are Plan F, Plan G, and High-Deductible Plan F. High-Deductible Plan F is not offered by all insurance companies, but it may represent quite a bargain. The cost sharing mechanism is different than the other plans. If you purchase a High-Deductible Plan F, then you are responsible for the first $2070 of costs. That amount is set annually by the CMS.

However, once you have met this deductible, then the High-Deductible Plan F will pay for all costs. There are no further copays or coinsurance. In addition, the Part B Excess will also be paid by this policy.

Is this a deal? That depends. If you have outstanding health (no medications, annual doctor's visits for maintenance), and are at an advanced age, then the answer could be yes. High-Deductible Plan F puts an absolute cap on your medical costs (except prescriptions). If you have financial difficulty but want "disaster insurance," then this may be a better use of money, compared to Medicare Advantage, because it covers the Medicare Part B Excess. You will need to calculate the annual premium, and compare it to the alternatives. The way to evaluate this is to divide the deductible by 12, the number of months, and then add that number (let's call it X), to the premium of the high-deductible Plan F. For 2012, the deductible is $2,070 so X = $172.50. Add that to the high-deductible Plan F premium, which is approximately $70/month for a 75-year-old. So, the total of $242.50 is the absolute worst case scenario. In this case, it is more probably the case that you experience some type of Part B excess change. That will be paid for by the high-deductible Plan F.

Medigap Open Enrollment During Q4?

This is a very specific situation, and should only be used with the cooperation of a knowledgeable agent. For those enrolling in Medigap for the first time during the last three months of the year, you can take advantage of the calendar. First, you should enroll in Plan F. The reason? You do not have to pay for the Part B deductible. That way, you can get not only the preventative care examination, which is free, but you can also receive any follow-up treatments, and the Medigap policy will pay for potential out-of-pocket expenses.

Pitfalls to Avoid When Choosing a Medigap Policy

Pre-Existing Condition Waiting Period

This quote is from "Choosing a Medigap Policy: A Guide to Health Insurance for People with Medicare" from the Centers for Medicare & Medicaid Services (CMS). "Remember, for Medicare covered services, original Medicare will still cover the condition, even if the Medigap policy won't cover your out-of-pocket costs, but you're responsible for the coinsurance or copayment."

BUT, Insurance Companies CAN Impose a Waiting Period

Again the source of this information is the Centers for Medicare & Medicaid Services. "While the insurance company can't make you wait for your coverage to start, it may be able to make you wait for coverage related to a pre-existing condition. A preexisting condition is a health problem you have before the date a new insurance policy starts. In some cases, the Medigap insurance company can refuse to cover your out-of-pocket costs for these pre-existing health problems for up to 6 months. This is called a 'pre-existing condition waiting period.' After 6 months, the Medigap policy will cover the pre-existing condition. Coverage for a pre-existing condition can only be excluded in a Medigap policy if the condition was treated or diagnosed within 6 months before the date the coverage starts under the Medigap policy. This is called the 'look-back period.'"

What This Means

If you are becoming Medicare eligible, then you have the right to choose any Medigap provider available in your state. However, after the 6 month Medigap open enrollment waiting period, then you may need to medically qualify (i.e. you may be asked questions about your medical situation).

Important note: If you have had creditable coverage continuously for the 6 months prior to Medicare eligibility, then no insurance company can deny you coverage under this stipulation.

It is important to NOT choose one that imposes the "pre-existing condition waiting period." If you want to know which companies these are, here is a HINT: find the companies that offer teaser rates. The teaser rate ends, there is a pre-existing waiting period, the waiting period ends, and then, in certain cases, you are unable to change providers.

Teaser Rates

If you are turning 65, then you are receiving teaser rates. You will receive a LOT of advertisements regarding Medicare Supplemental insurance (Medigap), the way that Medicare works, and different options. Often, you will receive lower initial monthly premiums. However, there are problems related to these low, initial prices.

You Can Change Medigap Carriers Anytime, UNLESS...

If you are unsatisfied with your Medigap insurance for any reason, you can change plans or companies at any time. However, if your health deteriorates, and you develop a medical condition, then you may be not be accepted by the new insurance company, because you may not be in your open enrollment period. Pre-existing conditions are not a factor during the open enrollment period ONLY. They may be a factor once out of the open enrollment period, depending upon the company, and the Medigap policy selected.

This happens.

A 65-year-old gentleman chooses a Medigap policy from a company with a low initial teaser-like rate. After two years, he is diagnosed with cancer. The low initial rate expires, and large rate increases occur. The man decides it is too expensive, but he may not be able to change Medigap policies. Now, the fact is that some companies MAY allow you to change, and some MAY NOT. You will need to check for yourself. Just be careful because the teaser rates may be too good to be true. However, this gentleman can switch to Medicare Advantage during the Annual Election Period.

This happens.

How to Avoid Pitfalls

Although there are no magic answers, here are some very good starting points.

First, eliminate companies that have the Medigap pre-existing condition waiting period. It makes no sense to become Medicare eligible, knowing that you require some treatment, and waiting for Medicare, just to have coverage by your Medigap policy denied during this waiting period. If your medical situation deteriorates during the first 6 months after enrolling in Medicare, and you require extensive medical attention immediately, then the amount not covered by Medicare Part A and Part B can be large. You will be liable for the cost sharing under original Medicare. Please remember that if you have had coverage for the 6 months prior to Medicare eligibility, this stipulation does not apply to you.

Second, you should ask an agent. You can distinguish an agent who has actual expertise of details by simply asking if the insurance company has the pre-existing condition waiting period. If the agent is unaware of the meaning of this waiting period (and there will be many who are unaware), then you need to find another agent. It isn't your job to educate the agent. It is your job to find an agent that you believe has full command of the details that can make a large difference to your welfare.

Third, ask an insurance company or an agent what price is being charged to current policyholders that are one year older than you are. For example let's say you are 67 years old and are considering changing from Medicare Advantage to Medigap, switching carriers, or switching Medigap plans with the same carrier. You can ask an insurance company or agent, "How much would the premium be if I were 68 years old?" The fact is that the price grids you are receiving in the mail may not be the rates that a current 68 year old policyholder is being charged. That is because the price grid may be a grid of introductory rates. There is no guarantee, of course, that the rate of increase will be the same in the future as it has been in the past. That said, insurance companies must justify rate increases by proving a Medical Loss Ratio (MLR). In fact, as of August 2012, insurance companies have been required to issue refunds if claims did not represent a ratio of premiums (less regulatory costs).

Fourth, avoid insurance companies that accept high-risk patients. Admittedly, we are wading out of the shallow end of the pool here. While all insurance companies must accept you during your Medigap open enrollment period, insurance companies may deny enrollment if you have a preexisting medical condition. Nevertheless, some companies may accept you. If you do not have a preexisting medical condition, but want to change to a Medigap policy, or to change your carrier for any reason, then you should select a company that denies coverage to those that do have a preexisting medical condition.

Why is this? The reason is that your future premiums are more likely to rise at a faster rate in the future if you purchase a Medigap policy from a company that does not place restrictions on enrollment. Insurance companies can raise prices based on the claims history of the other policy owners that have the same policy. Therefore, there is no reason to enroll in a policy and be in the same pool with others that are more likely to have a greater incidence of claims, because those higher claims will justify higher premiums in the future. Before merely choosing a Medigap policy from a carrier that charges the lowest price, this deserves careful consideration because you may be not be able to switch Medigap carriers in the future, and will then be subject to its future rate increases.

Table 4. Medigap Plans

How to read the chart: If a check mark appears in a column of this chart, the Medigap policy covers 100% of the described benefit. If a row lists a percentage, the policy covers that percentage of the described benefit. If a row is blank, the policy doesn't cover that benefit. **Note:** The Medigap policy covers coinsurance only after you have paid the deductible (unless the Medigap policy also covers the deductible).

Medigap Benefits	Medigap Plans									
	A	B	C	D	F*	G	K	L	M	N
Medicare Part A Coinsurance and hospital costs up to an additional 365 days after Medicare benefits are used up	✓	✓	✓	✓	✓	✓	✓	✓	✓	✓
Medicare Part B Coinsurance or Copayment	✓	✓	✓	✓	✓	✓	50%	75%	✓	✓***
Blood (First 3 Pints)	✓	✓	✓	✓	✓	✓	50%	75%	✓	✓
Part A Hospice Care Coinsurance or Copayment	✓	✓	✓	✓	✓	✓	50%	75%	✓	✓
Skilled Nursing Facility Care Coinsurance			✓	✓	✓	✓	50%	75%	✓	✓
Medicare Part A Deductible		✓	✓	✓	✓	✓	50%	75%	50%	✓
Medicare Part B Deductible			✓		✓					
Medicare Part B Excess Charges					✓	✓				
Foreign Travel Emergency (Up to Plan Limits)			✓	✓	✓	✓				✓
							Out-of-Pocket Limit**			
							$4,660	$2,330		

*Plan F also offers a high-deductible plan. If you choose this option, this means you must pay for Medicare-covered costs up to the deductible amount of $2,070 in 2012 before your Medigap plan pays anything.

**After you meet your out-of-pocket yearly limit and your yearly Part B deductible ($147 in 2012), the Medigap plan pays 100% of covered services for the rest of the calendar year.

***Plan N pays 100% of the Part B coinsurance, except for a copayment of up to $20 for some office visits and up to a $50 copayment for emergency room visits that don't result in an inpatient admission.

Source: CMS

Chapter 7. Employer-Sponsored Group Plans

This chapter focuses on the retiree from a company after many years of service and on active employees that are eligible for Medicare. Often times there is a employer-sponsored group plan which includes health insurance, maybe life insurance, as well as some other benefits, such as dental and vision.

There are many reasons that an employer-provided retiree health insurance plan can be inferior to the private market. First, you must understand that insurance companies themselves are not interested in providing group plans for persons who are Medicare eligible. As a person who arranges employer-sponsored health insurance plans, I can see the pricing for persons who are Medicare eligible, and it is much more expensive for persons to have group plans then to have an individual Medicare plan. Second, employers do not want to bear the additional and ever-rising costs associated with retiree health insurance. Employers understand that the Medicare system is fundamentally going to be challenged over time, and employers are, in general, in no position to pay the rising costs with no end in sight. This is particularly true for those companies that have downsized significantly, and whose number of retirees is larger than that of active employees. Increasing life expectancy has only made the situation more drastic from the employer's point of view. When you add up these concerns, then it is no wonder that the cost sharing terms of employer-sponsored plans are eroding. The degree at which they are changing differs widely among employers, but there is little doubt that this is occurring.

Pay Careful Attention to Enrollment Issues

Warning on Employer-Sponsored Enrollment Calendar

Special care is required regarding the election periods when an employer-sponsored group plan is involved. The reason? Employer-sponsored group plans frequently have different enrollment periods than Medicare. For example, many large employer-sponsored group plans have enrollment periods that end after Medicare's Annual Election Period (AEP, October 15 – December 7). Procrastinators have made, are making, and will make the error of waiting until the last moment before deciding upon the right configuration of benefits (group vs Medicare, etc). If you wait too long, the selection can be made for you. Worse yet, both the Annual Election Period and the employer-sponsored group plan enrollment period end, and you are left with original Medicare. Be careful.

Check the Medicare Enrollment Requirement

The saying goes, "The devil is in the details." This old cliché exists for a reason. Here is a prime example of why. In most employer-sponsored retiree group plans, you will have to pay for your Medicare Part B premium which is the $104.90 a month for 2013. You must check this yourself, because that will greatly determine whether or not it is a good idea to continue on with your employee group plan. **DO NOT ASSUME ANYTHING: there are many cases when the Human Resources department does not inform employees/retirees whether they are required to enroll in Medicare Part B.** If your employer-sponsored plan requires you to enroll in Medicare Part B, and you do not, then the monthly premiums that you pay to your employer-sponsored plan will most likely be entirely worthless. That is because Medicare is the primary insurer, and the group plan is the secondary insurer. In this example, there is no primary insurer.

It is very important to know the cost sharing arrangement of your retiree health plan. You have received a book every year, most likely one which is a Summary of Benefits. It will tell you the schedule of the deductibles, coinsurance, as well as copayments under different medical situations.

This happens.

An employee, currently 67 years old, is in excellent health when he becomes eligible for Medicare Part B at 65 years old. He doesn't read the employee benefits package he has received, so he doesn't enroll in Medicare Part B. Now, at 67 years old, he requires extensive medical attention. He finds out that his retiree benefits require enrollment in Medicare Part B, which has not elected. His retiree benefits are null and void, premiums have been deducted from his pension already, he will need to enroll in Medicare Part B, and will have a penalty for 4 years, i.e. twice the length of time that he was eligible for Medicare Part B, but did not enroll.

This happens.

Examine Cost Sharing Terms Carefully

Check the Premium

The easiest, and first, step is to check the total premium that will be deducted from your pension plan check. In addition to knowing the Medicare Part B enrollment rules, you also need to know the group plan's enrollment rules. Can you cancel at any time during the year, or are you required to enroll for the entire calendar year? Can you change your mind, and when?

Every employer has a different combination. There is no way to generalize.

Check the Co-Pay, Coinsurance and Annual Out-of-Pocket Maximum

This is also easy. The key things to focus on are: cost of office visits, emergency room costs, and annual deductible. You must understand how much you will pay if you are admitted to the hospital. Is this an annual amount, or is it an amount per benefit period? Finally, is there a maximum amount, above which the employer-sponsored plan pays 100%? Lastly, you can check to see if the retiree group plan will cover the Part B Excess defined earlier in this book. Most likely, the Medicare Excess is not covered at all under retiree group health insurance plans.

One additional point: some group retiree plans have different copay schedules for office visits. It is a trend for retiree group plans to charge different rates for specialists, and some retiree group plans do not cover specialist visits at all. That means urologists for men, and gynecologists for women. It would be wise to check this carefully. Note that this is part of the preventative care visit, which is free annually in accordance with the Patient Protection and Affordable Care Act. Medicare Advantage is inconsistent with respect to this. Medigap does not distinguish ($20 per office visit). But in many cases, group plans do. This can be a hidden out-of-pocket cost for group retirees (and their spouses).

Prescription Coverage

Again, this is an entirely mixed bag. Every company will have their own plan with respect to prescriptions. You can most likely see that there is a copay schedule for generic and non-generic prescriptions. You should check to see if there is an annual deductible. Finally, you should find out if there is a Coverage Gap ("donut hole"). Just because it is a group plan, do not assume that the group plan has no donut hole for the Medicare-eligible. Some employer-sponsored plans have no Coverage Gap, and some do. It is conceivable to change prescription coverage within the same "group plan" when you become Medicare-eligible.

Married, Group Coverage, and Medicare: Who Pays First?

The primary factor here will be price. In certain cases, the price of the combined insurance will be low enough to justify the risk. That is entirely up to you, your financial resources, and your comfort in believing that you will remain healthy over a long period of time. If you are married and have group coverage, then the group coverage and Medicare will work together to a large degree. However, that is the case anyway, when you have either a Medicare Advantage or Medigap plan. Therefore, the point is not that they collaborate with each other, the point is to figure out, if you are married, how to cover both people in the least expensive, most complete way possible.

It isn't impossible to figure this out, but it is close. It is probably not a good idea to try to remember all of these configurations; just find the one that applies to you, and ignore the rest. Here are the rules, and there are many exceptions, depending on whether you have a specific medical condition (such as Black Lung, or End-Stage Renal Disease).

Large Employer (>100 employees)	
Spouse works, and You are covered under spouse	Group first, Medicare second
Spouse works, You are disabled and covered under spouse	Group first, Medicare second
Small Employer (< 100 employees)	
Spouse works, and You are covered under spouse	Medicare first, group second
Spouse works, You are disabled and covered under spouse	Medicare first, group second

Exceptions:

End Stage Renal Disease	
First 30 months of Medicare entitlement	Group health first, Medicare second
After first 30 months of Medicare entitlement	Medicare first, Group health second
End Stage Renal Disease and COBRA	
First 30 months of Medicare entitlement	COBRA first, Medicare second
After first 30 months of Medicare entitlement	Medicare first, COBRA second

Source: CMS, "Medicare and Other Health Benefits: Your Guide to Who Pays First"

If you have read the above, and are not confused, then you are in the vast minority. However, a couple of points apply to ALL of the above conditions. First, it isn't clear how much of any given treatment the "second" insurer will pay. Second, it also is not clear how much, if any, of the Medicare Part B Excess Charges that the "second" insurer will pay. That is total guesswork, and for that reason alone, it is still my recommendation that you should consider dropping group coverage in favor of an independent plan (Medicare Advantage or Medigap). The last thing that you want is for your cost sharing arrangement to be a mystery. If you are a patient, the priority should be on GETTING HEALTHIER, not on wondering/worrying about your out-of-pocket expenses. This doesn't mean that neither a Medicare Advantage nor a Medigap plan would be best; the recommendation here is to see what your group plan doesn't explicitly state, and ask questions about it. From there, you will know what risks remain, and decide if you are comfortable with that risk.

Employer-Sponsored Medicare Advantage

When you become Medicare eligible, it is vital to know what plan the employer is providing to you. It can be the case that the employer is enrolling you in a Medicare Advantage plan whose network may not be the same as the plan you were using prior to Medicare eligibility. The confusing part of this is that the Medicare plan that you were given as a retiree can be different fundamentally from the HMO or PPO that you have been given as an active employee in your pre-Medicare days. That means that the list of providers may or may not be the same providers that covered you before you were Medicare eligible. This is a very important point, and as a result you need to consider carefully what you are actually doing, and what you were actually electing. If you travel out of the state frequently, or for many months during the year, you can end up finding out that your total medical costs, meaning your premiums plus out-of-pocket expenses, may exceed other arrangements which could be done in the private market, where there may be no such restrictions.

The General Case

For many persons, the employer-sponsored retiree plan is the best plan. The overriding reason may be price. In certain cases, retirees are not required to pay for the Medicare Part B premium. In certain cases, there is no donut hole, as mentioned in an earlier chapter. If this is the case, then the employer-sponsored plan may be a better way to go. Your total cost of protection may be lower under an employer-sponsored group plan, even if that means that there are unfavorable copayments and deductibles.

However, none of this solves the dilemma. The terms and conditions of your plan can change without notice and without your input.

The problem with this is that your total cost can increase if your copayment and deductible schedules all increase, and you will have no control over it. This will be governed under the agreement between the employer and the insurance company.

Let's take some real-life examples.

This section is intentionally left blank.

This Happens: A Bankrupt Company

There is a company under the auspices of the Pension Benefit Guaranty Corporation (PBGC); I will call it just company D. It offers a group plan for retirees, which is similar to that of a Medigap as well as a prescription drug plan, and this company requires enrollees to pay for Medicare Part B. The prescription drug plan has the same provisions as Medicare Part D, which means that it also includes a coverage gap. The employer also charges a monthly premium which includes both the drug as well as the medical plan.

In combination with each other, the problem here is that the total cost of the additional amounts charged on a monthly basis, on top of the Part B deductible, begins at $160 a month. In this particular case, the medical coverage is no better than what exists in the Medigap market. To summarize, the coverage is no better, AND the price is higher. It is both more expensive, and provides fewer benefits. Nevertheless, retirees stay with this disadvantageous plan. It is incredible, but true.

This happens.

This section is intentionally left blank.

> ### *This Happens: A Global, Thriving Company*
>
> Often times the reason an employer-sponsored retiree benefit plan may seem cheaper is due to the fact that the employer has put in money from its own funds in order to keep the prices low, to the benefit of its retirees. However, the employer may not be under the obligation to do so, and it can discontinue this type of subsidy if the funds that it has reserved for this purpose have been depleted. To make matters worse, legacy collective bargaining agreements, due to mergers and acquisitions, have restricted companies from renegotiating costly retiree health benefit plans.
>
> If this is the case, premiums may increase substantially. In fact, you can look in financial statements, or in the small print of the Summary of Benefits you have been given. A description of your summary of benefits may well describe a situation where the company can choose to discontinue the subsidy and increases are passed to the retiree. The net effect of this type of employer-sponsored retiree group plan is that the benefits are no better than that that exists in the private market, and the costs may be no better, and in certain cases can be more expensive than insurance that exists in the private market.
>
> This situation is real and many persons who have been dedicated employees to a particular employer for a long period of time may be disappointed. But given the pressures on treasury departments of large corporations, this can easily be the case.
>
> *This happens.*

Medicare-Eligible Retiree & Non-Medicare-Eligible Spouse

There are certain situations where you will need to stay with your employer-sponsored group plan, even if it is more expensive, and your cost sharing terms are worse than is available under a Medicare Advantage or Medigap plan. The primary situation is when the retiree is married to a non-Medicare eligible person. Most (the large majority) group plans do not allow a retiree to disenroll and keep the spouse on the employer-sponsored plan.

If that is the case, then the question is going to be whether or not the spouse is eligible for private health insurance. If the spouse cannot obtain private health insurance, then you may have no other choice than to stay with the group plan.

If your spouse can obtain private health insurance, then you need to see how the numbers might actually work together. It will most likely be the case that the spouse can obtain health insurance at a cheaper rate than the price being charged by the employer. The reason for this is that a spouse is charged more than the employee in group plans. It works this way to prevent people staying in their jobs simply to obtain health insurance for his/her spouse.

Dental, Vision, and Other "Benefits"

Some retirees believe that there are other types of additional benefits as part of the employer-sponsored plan which are very important, such as dental and vision insurance. However, the reality is that dental and vision insurance is often times very limited. These types of insurance are limited; benefits are very low, unless you use the entire maximum benefit every year. It is very frequently the case that you will be able to find the dental and vision coverage which is at least as good as the employer-sponsored plan. For those persons that require extensive dental work, for example, you will find that the annual benefit amounts can be somewhere in the $1500-$1000 per year per person. As a result, the amount of benefit actually received by the retiree and their family members is very limited. Private-market vision and dental can frequently be obtained for cheaper prices than is being charged by employer-sponsored plans. It is simply more convenient for you to select the "package deal." It is costing you money that you would otherwise use for better health insurance or prescription drug coverage.

If Your Employer Cancels Retiree Health Benefits

It can be the case that an employer simply stops providing retiree health benefits. This has happened, this is happening (and being actively considered), and it will happen. There can be little or no warning in advance. You probably know someone that has received this type of notification in the mail. This is what to do.

First, do not panic. You will be allowed to select an Medicare Advantage or a Medigap plan, along with a Medicare Part D plan, if necessary, under a Special Election Period (SEP). From the date of discontinuation, you will have 63 days to select a new plan, without incurring a penalty.

Second, you will need to keep the copy of the notice of cancellation from your employer and/or the insurance company that provided the employer-sponsored health benefits. In your Summary of Benefits, or in a separate document, there will be a Letter of Creditable Coverage. This will be necessary to use as evidence of your eligibility for the SEP.

Third, you will most likely be directed by your employer to a particular plan or company as a substitute. **You should not sign up on the spot, without checking the market first.** Remember that the sponsor of the meeting, the employer, is the same one that is discontinuing your coverage. The employer is doing what is best for its constituents, its shareholders/owners. You should do the same, and act for yourself. You have a constituency as well: yourself, your family, and those that care about you.

This happens.

Globally recognized company has declared bankruptcy during the early 2000s. Salaried employees, not protected from bankruptcy, have employee benefits slowly, but inevitably, taken from them. Finally, retiree health benefits are next. Medicare-eligible white-collar workers are given a stipend as a substitute for health benefits, and they attend coordinated employee information sessions. Many employees accept the recommendations, and enroll in the Medigap policy presented during these sessions. Now, that insurance company faces severe claims experience, and rates have gone up multiple times a year. Those with preexisting conditions are largely ineligible from switching to other carriers (insurance companies), because the open enrollment period is over, and the Special Election Period has also expired. The retiree now can choose to either accept rapidly rising premiums, or a plan with less-complete coverage.

This happens.

You can freely select any MA or MAPD during this period. You can freely select any Prescription Drug Plan during this period. However, you may or may not be able to select a specific Medigap plan. There will be some selection allowed, but it may be the case that all insurance companies do not offer all plans to you. Therefore, if you have a specific plan in mind, then you will need to check around. Do not accept information from outside sources if they tell you it is completely impossible to purchase a particular plan. Different companies have made different business decisions regarding this.

Insurance companies have differing policies when applicants attempt to enroll in Medigap. This is an important, overlooked fact. Some people just think that they will deal with the issue if the employer cancels coverage, or if the cost sharing arrangement dramatically changes. Well, when it occurs, you may have wanted a particular Medigap plan. Depending upon the insurance company, this option may not be available to you at that time. You may then look back, with regret, for not taking matters into your own hands, especially if the financial aspects were roughly equal. And you know what? You could have done something about it then, and now you will face an uncertain health and financial outcome, as a result of not addressing this issue when it was within your control. The point of this book is to help you to avoid this situation, and all other situations where the outcome is handed to you. The point of this book is to help you take control of your healthcare expenses, and your household's well-being (health, emotional, and financial).

Medigap Restructuring Has Occurred and May Happen Again

No one will be surprised if Medicare changes, and not for the better, in the future. Certain aspects of certain Medigap plans are being examined, because they expose the Medicare system to abuse, by both patients and providers. This notion comes from a journalist on the KaiserHealthNews.org website (an excellent resource) in the article entitled, "Health Law Prompts Review Of Some Medigap Plans; Defining Who Gets Dependent Status" on August 12, 2012. Indeed, certain Medigap plans have been discontinued in the past. Existing policyholders have continued on with their policies as originally conceived. However, there are no new enrollees allowed into the discontinued plans.

Well, given that Medicare is being examined, and that it is well-established that fundamental changes may be in order over time, it is reasonable to presume that certain plans may not be available in the future. Let's take the situation in which you wanted superior coverage, but planned to change "when I get older." Now, that day has arrived. What if the plan that you wanted doesn't exist? Was it worth it? That will be left to you to decide. However, given that extreme medical costs are one of the two most important potentially catastrophic financial events that can occur to a household, you should consider this very, very carefully. You will be accepting a risk that could result in costs that jeopardize not only yourself, but those around you as well. If the premium amounts are equivalent, then this is a "no-brainer." If you look carefully, it is very likely that you will be able to find plans which are slightly more expensive, and provide far better coverage. Anecdotally, the error that can be seen the most is when someone tries to save $10 per month on premium. The weaker coverage ends up costing that person thousands of dollars, annually. It is much worse than that, because there is also the doubt about the future on top of the actual extra financial costs. Maybe it would have been wiser to forego one bottle of wine a month, and secure you and your family's physical, emotional, and financial well-being.

What Employers Can Do

This topic is too broad to cover in one section. It will be the topic of another book by itself. However, there are some guidelines to follow. First, both employers and employees can be better off if employers create incentives for employees to elect a Medicare plan or Medigap plan independently. This may require negotiation of existing contracts. Nevertheless, the savings will be well worth it. Second, the employer-sponsored group plan should provide for those whose families require group coverage, because there will be cases in which family members cannot otherwise obtain health insurance at a reasonable price. Third, health savings accounts (HSA) are a good way to incentive employees to maintain their health, and to lower costs. They can be established so that if people need to defer election of Medicare Part B, then that person may be able to save extra money, on a pre-tax basis, which can be used to pay for Medicare Part B premiums when he/she enrolls in Medicare Part B. One of the group health plan alternatives should include a High Deductible Health Plan, which works alongside with Health Savings Accounts.

Objections that employees or retirees may raise can be solved by one of three suggestions. Sometimes, collective bargaining tensions prevent reasonableness by all parties. However, if employer and employees work together, the difference in pricing between group plans and Medicare plans is so large that the cost savings are worth the effort. There are many instances, however, when the rational solution remains elusive. Employer / employee relations become strained, reasonableness is not considered, and both sides suffer. These days, this can be easily found in the case of municipalities, where fiscal concerns are clashing with legacy collective bargaining agreements.

This happens.

Unionized employees and their employer, a local government under financial duress, are renegotiating their collective bargaining agreement. The agreement stipulates that retirees are entitled to identical coverage that they received when they were active employees. Now, Medicare Advantage and Medigap are superior in both price and coverage to the benefits they were receiving when these retirees were active employees. However, the union and management cannot find a middle ground, and the active employees go on strike.

This happens.

For employers, the cost savings can be large enough to ensure the viability of a business/company. For employees, not only are the prices lower, but the coverage is often superior to that offered by a group plan. Perhaps we can all agree on one thing: an employer choosing to close his/her business due to the high cost of health insurance is the least favorable outcome. Those are the stakes. As such, everything should be explored fully. If you are an employer, and you have Medicare-eligible employees or retirees, then you should actively attempt to find a better solution. More than likely, you will be successful in finding one.

One solution, a very good one, is being adopted by a few selected large employers. They are adopting Medigap High-Deductible Plan F for everyone that is Medicare eligible, and allowing their retirees to pay for additional amounts of insurance. As a reminder, High-Deductible Plan F is a Medigap policy that has a large deductible ($2070 in 2012), and the Medicare beneficiary pays it. Thereafter there are no further copays or deductibles. Certain clever employers are providing a cost sharing agreement of this $2070 with retirees. For example, the retiree pays $50 per month but then only has to pay a maximum of $1000 per year, and the employer covers $1070. Now, the High-Deductible Plan F is satisfied. If claims are above this, then the Medigap High-Deductible Plan F pays for the remainder. *This is entirely possible and an excellent solution* for both employers and Medicare-eligible retirees. Difficult times require creativity, and this is indeed creative.

Chapter 8. Special Groups

Veterans Administration (VA)

As you may know, Veterans Administration benefits, including retiree health benefits, is a very complicated matter. There are benefits as well as drawbacks to the VA medical system for those who are eligible for Medicare.

The most comprehensive set is called Tricare For Life (TFL), for those persons who have been in the military as a career; they are entitled to a full set of benefits. In addition, it has been the case that those persons that suffered a disability that is directly linked to active combat may also be granted TFL. The most prevalent case is when someone has a documented case of exposure to Agent Orange, and has suffered from a medical situation that has been linked to that exposure. In other cases, it is not granted. The best way to find out if you are entitled to TFL is to contact the Veterans Administration.

This section presumes that a veteran knows how to register in the Defense Enrollment Eligibility Reporting System, otherwise known as DEERS (http://tricare.mil/mybenefit/home/overview/Eligibility/DEERS) or the Department of Veteran Affairs website (http://va.gov/healthbenefits/online).

To use your Tricare For Life, your military identification will identify you as a TFL beneficiary. As a result of it, you will have some small co-pays for your prescriptions and you will also have complete medical coverage. That medical coverage is based on the military set of approved procedures and treatments. Please note: the list of approved procedures and treatments is NOT identical to Medicare-approved procedures and treatments. They are separate, but clearly, there is substantial overlap. A particular treatment belonging to TFL's approved therapies and not belonging to Medicare's approved treatments is very rare, but there are instances in which this peculiar situation does exist.

As long as you are your treatments are on the TFL-approved list of procedures and treatments, then you are fully covered. You will have to enroll in Medicare Part A and Part B. There will be some procedures that are approved by Medicare, but not approved by TFL. If this is the case, then you will need to pay the deductible and copays as per Medicare rules.

There are public policy questions regarding TFL. You may be aware of this; Congress has debated whether or not TFL should remain free, and/or whether or not TFL should be administered by the private sector. Those questions remain open, and are beyond the scope of this book.

If you are not entitled to TFL, you still may qualify for VA benefits. You will need to individually enroll. You can do this online by applying at: https://www.1010ez.med.va.gov/. For those that qualify, an individualized set of benefits is awarded according to eight separate tiers. The VA will determine which tier you belong to. That is beyond the scope of this book. Some aspects are shared in common by most, if not all, eight tiers. Here is a list of some, but not all of those aspects.

You will be assigned a primary care provider and will need to attend VA facilities, which exist nationwide. For some, this is acceptable. For others, it isn't practical, because VA facilities are not in the vicinity. VA benefits generally provide prescriptions benefits at very reasonable costs, comparable to Medicare Part D. The extent of the benefits that you receive can be subject to review. From this perspective, one should be careful.

> **This happens.**
>
> Eligibility and cost sharing is subject to review by the VA. Please know that if you have been receiving VA benefits in the past, it may not necessarily be the case in the future. If you eligibility is examined, the opposite can also occur. It has been the case that a person that was previously receiving limited benefits from the VA has been stripped of these benefits, which left the Medicare-eligible beneficiary in a position in which he had to find both health insurance and prescription insurance.
>
> *This happens.*

If you do not qualify for TFL, and yet are eligible to receive prescriptions through VA services, there are a couple of things to know. The first is that insulin is usually not well covered by VA benefits. This may be a reason to purchase the cheapest possible MAPD or a stand-alone prescription plan (Medicare Part D). The second is that if you solely use VA medical facilities and do not require a prescription drug plan, then you have a special situation. Earlier, the idea of "additional benefits" was described as part of certain MA and/or MAPD plans. An easy example would be that there may be discounts for smoking cessation programs.

Within MA, there are certain plans that have zero ($0) premium. They are without prescription benefits, which is fine since you may receive your prescriptions through the VA. A VA beneficiary can get a zero premium plan, use the additional benefits, and use VA facilities for medical services and VA pharmacies for prescriptions. As of this writing, there is NO CONFLICT in this setup. Additionally, you can use the MA card (although there will be cost sharing in accordance with the MA or MAPD plan) if you strongly prefer to not use VA facilities. If you have an "emergency" that is not ruled to qualify as an "emergency," then you would have a lower out-of-pocket cost by using your Medicare Advantage plan.

This happens.

A VA beneficiary goes to the emergency room at local hospital, which is not a VA hospital, with the belief that he is very ill. It turns out to be nothing. He has to pay the full cost of the services administered at the emergency room. The only portion that is reimbursed is the ambulance transfer from the non-VA facility to the VA facility, and then only if coordinated by the VA facility.

This happens.

If you do qualify for TFL, then you can also benefit from this same arrangement. You can enroll in a zero premium plan, and choose the plan that has "additional benefits" that accompany the MA or MAPD, and reap the additional benefits that may be offered with that MA/MAPD plan, free of charge. That's right. Free.

You may wonder, "How does this work?" or "How is this possible?" The reason is that under MA or MAPD, the Medicare system hands the processing of claims, the accounting of claims, etc to the private insurance company. The Medicare system pays the private insurance company a lot of money to take the place of CMS. The individual uses some of this money in order to pay for the extra benefits, under the idea that these extra benefits will result in better health, and therefore lower medical claims.

Federal Employee Health Benefits (FEHB) Program

Eligible persons include both active employees and retirees from the U.S. Federal Government, including U.S. Postal Service employees and retirees. If you are Medicare-eligible, then you have a couple of difficult choices, and it does depend on whether or not you are federal government employee/retiree or a Postal Service employee/retiree.

Enrollment in the FEHB runs on a different calendar than the Medicare Annual Election Period.

Federal government employees/retirees have comprehensive health and prescription coverage. There is no donut hole in the FEHB program. In addition, persons under FEHB can elect an MA/MAPD in addition to their existing benefits, and there is no conflict. In short, it is the same as if a person is entitled to Tricare For Life as described earlier. Even if you stay with the FEHB, you can subscribe to a zero premium MA/MAPD, and reap the additional benefits that may be offered with that MA/MAPD plan, free of charge. That's correct: there are some MA plans with no premium.

FEHB for normal enrollees do face an issue, however. That issue is price. For federal government employees, the most comprehensive plan is expensive when compared to the private market for similar coverage, except for the donut hole. The bottom line is that if you are in excellent health, then it might be prudent to choose a more affordable plan with little or no change in coverage.

Postal Service employees face a different set of circumstances. As of the current writing, the premium charged to Postal Service employees is far lower, and cannot be replicated in the private market. For postal employees, the zero premium MA/MAPD plan, in conjunction with FEHB Plan benefits, will result in the lowest cost, along with the additional benefits that can sometimes be offered with MA/MAPD plans. If you are married, spouses of Postal Service employees need to be considered. Spouses of postal services employees are charged at different rates from the employee. If the spouse of a Postal Employee is Medicare-eligible, then all of the statements regarding group insurance apply. In short, Medicare and a Medicare Advantage/Medigap plan may be a better setup. That may depend upon the Part D Coverage Gap ("donut hole"), i.e. if the spouse of a Postal Service employee/retiree requires large amounts of prescriptions, then staying inside the FEHB Plan may be best.

This happens.

Active postal service employee is married to a Medicare-eligible spouse. The spouse elects to not enroll in Medicare Part B when she turned 65 years old. However, over the course of the next year, she develops a medical situation, and her husband retires before turning 65 years old. The human resources representative informs the employee that he and his spouse will no longer be eligible for FEHB benefits. The spouse enrolls in Medicare under a Special Election Period (SEP). However, the issue is the she cannot choose the Medigap plan that would have been cheapest, and must choose the next best alternative, when she could have selected her initial choice if she had enrolled in Medicare when she was first eligible.

This happens.

This section is intentionally left blank.

> **This happens.**
>
> A retired Federal government employee has the retiree plan through the U.S. government. The FEHB program allows for a Medicare Advantage plan in addition to Medicare Part B and the group plan provided to retirees. She enrolls, so that she can benefit from the "extras" that are included with the Medicare Advantage plan, which has no premium. Upon visiting the physician, the billing manager at the physician's office incorrectly tells her that there is a conflict of coverage. The billing manager is 100% wrong because she doesn't know this detail which is explicitly stated in the FEHB plan's Summary of Benefits. The retiree becomes worried, and unnecessarily cancels her no-premium Medicare Advantage plan, and is now ineligible to receive the extra benefits that accompany that Medicare Advantage plan.
>
> *This happens.*

State and Local Government Employees

State and local governments cannot be summarized in one easy phrase. All states and local governments (whether that be a city or county) have their own separate agreements.

State government employees may or may not be required to enroll in Medicare Part B when initially eligible. However, it is highly likely that you will be required to enroll in Medicare Part B. You will need to check that, and most states describe how Medicare will work with that state's health plan. You should ask the following questions. First, you will need to find out if Medicare Part B enrollment is required. Second, you will need to know how Medicare will work with your governmental plan. It is typically the case that Medicare will be the primary provider, and your state's plan will be secondary. Third, if Medicare is primary and your state's plan is secondary, then you will need to find out exactly what your state's plan will cover, above and beyond what original Medicare covers. Most plans do not specify whether or not the Part B Excess charge is paid by the government-sponsored plan. That is another way of saying, "No, but confirm this by yourselves." Finally, it would be a good idea to find out if you and disenroll from your government-sponsored plan and then re-enter at a later date. Again, it is unlikely this is the case, but you should know this before making a decision.

Local government contracts are usually quite different. Since there can be collective bargaining agreements for certain workers (sanitation, maintenance, transportation), it can be very delicate. Here are some important guidelines.

First, if your local government compensates you for "opting out," paying you cash in exchange for you cancelling your group plan, then you should examine this carefully. It may well be that this is worth it. That, of course, depends on whether you have a spouse that is not Medicare-eligible, and whether or not the spouse can remain in the group plan, if you decide to opt out.

Second, the terms and conditions of your benefits will vary widely from location to location. That will be the single biggest factor in deciding whether or not you should keep your retiree benefits plan. In the best cases, retiree benefits are continuing without any changes. In other cases, bankruptcy has been declared, and governments have tried to discontinue retiree health benefits entirely, as has been the case in Stockton, California (Los Angeles Times, 12 July 2012). If you stay in your group plan, then the price that will be deducted from your paycheck or pension may be too high. This is especially the case when you figure in the out-of-pocket expenses in conjunction with your group plan, and compare it to a Medicare Advantage or Medigap plan.

Third, you need to explore whether or not you can opt out of your medical and prescription coverage, and retain your dental and vision coverage. You should consider whether or not the price that you are charged for this dental and vision coverage is worth the price that you pay, when compared to the private market (see "Dental, Vision, and Other 'Benefits'" from the previous chapter).

A special type of employee is a public school educator. Faced with budgetary problems, state governments are being forced to change the benefits packages of both active and retired teachers. For example, in the State of Michigan, a new motion has been passed to enact this. The result of this is that retired teachers have been faced with a changing landscape regarding their retiree health benefits. In many cases, new teachers will face a future without retiree health benefits. For currently retired teachers, higher premiums may result. The point of this is that teachers may need to look at prices, because the price in the private market may soon approach the retiree benefits package's price. The nature of the group has changed, but the message is the same: educators will not be able to simply presume that their retiree benefits package is the best that they can afford.

Unions

"If your friend jumped off a bridge, would you follow him/her?" – Parent to child
"I will stay with my group plan. My buddies say that everything has worked out OK." -Same person commenting about his group benefits under Medicare

In coffee shops around the country, you can hear this conversation. That is guaranteed. This section addresses employees and retirees that are members of unions governed by collective bargaining agreements. This section does not include hourly UAW auto workers, who are covered by the Retiree Benefits Trust, a VEBA trust. Unfortunately, the bottom line is you will face many of the same things that other Medicare-eligible employees face. Most times, union contracts heavily favor active employees. I am certain that you have already faced this.

Union officials have motivations to promote group plans. One primary reason is that group pricing may be dependent upon the number of enrollees in the retiree group plan, or the percentage of enrollment. While that may be admirable for the group as a whole, the problem is that it may not be good for the individual, i.e. you.

What this means is that if you have a medical situation, you are back to my base case. You need to fend for yourself. Examine for yourself, investigate for yourself, and ultimately, decide for yourself. Unless the collective bargaining agreement has closed down the Medicare Part D coverage gap, and you or your spouse require medications that exceed Medicare Part D coverage, the almost-inevitable conclusion will be that an individual plan, whether that is a Medicare Advantage or a Medigap policy along with a standalone prescription drug plan, will be more cost effective.

The recommendations that I am making here may seem controversial, because as part of a union, you probably have friends and colleagues who are roughly your age. Those friends or colleagues have gone through the Medicare system. The main piece of advice to leave with you is to not generalize their situation to yours, and don't presume that just because things have worked out well for a longtime friend, that it fits your individual situation. That is probably the wrong approach because every person's health situation can be different, their sensitivities can be different, and their financial situation can be different. In other words, just because your friend jumped off a bridge doesn't necessarily mean that it is a good idea for you. The choices you make (or not) can drain your household net worth either as a one-time event, or on an ongoing basis. As close as you may have been with your friend or colleague for many years, that does not mean that they have the same experiences you have. Now, you may think this is obvious, right? You would be shocked at the frequency that this is the answer given to agents and advisors.

Finding out the information for yourself, and making an informed, intentional choice is the best path. Life may or may not work out as you envisioned; hopefully, it is better than you have hoped. However, the intent of this book is to avoid taking risks that you did not intend. That is not to say that life is riskless, it isn't. That is not the same thing as you choosing the risks that you are willing to accept, and avoiding those that you do not want to accept. You may have financial reasons for choosing a particular plan. You have deeply private motivations. It isn't the goal of this book to cast judgment on your motivations. However, using the information presented here, you can accept risks with full, or nearly full, information.

Hospital (and Other Healthcare) Employees

Separately, I want to address employees of healthcare organizations, such as hospitals, nursing homes, or home health care service organizations. For personnel who work at hospitals, or home healthcare services, it is sad and disappointing to report that the health benefits available at these organizations can be no better than your average group employer in an industry unrelated to health. In fact, healthcare organizations frequently discontinue health insurance entirely once a person becomes inactive.

In hospitals you may know that active employees can work beyond the age of 65. Those persons are generally covered. The issue for you is that if you are Medicare eligible, you must check your benefits very carefully when you turn 65. Different organizations offer a wide range of alternatives. You may need to sign up for Medicare Part B, or you may not be required to sign up for Part B. You may have your choice. You can read the section

107

titled "Married, Group coverage, and Medicare: Who Pays First? Good Luck." You will need to refer to it again. Healthcare providers vary widely in size, so you will need to carefully read to identify your situation.

One special provision can accompany group coverage for hospital employees: prescription drugs are often offered to hospital employees at substantial discounts. These discounts, if combined with the lack of Coverage Gap, can represent substantially lower out-of-pocket expenses for those on large amounts of prescriptions.

Small Business Owners

This section is geared to the small business owner. At the end of Chapter 7, there is a section called "What Employers Can Do." The issues and challenges stated in that section are ones that should be very familiar to the small business owner. In addition to the issues mentioned in that chapter, there are additional challenges that need to be faced, since the business owner is the main stakeholder, there may be legal, tax, and accounting issues, all of which are ultimately the responsibility of the owner. Depending upon the size and scope of the business, you may require an outside advisor. From a health insurance perspective, a Medicare-eligible small business owner should keep a few things in mind.

The new regulations that index your Medicare Part B and Part D premiums to income are complicating matters for high-income earners. Since Medicare Part B and Part D are indexed to your annual income, it may be that the cost of the premiums is as high as your small business group health insurance premium. For example, if you make over $214,000 a year, then your monthly Part B premium will be $319.80 a month. When you add a Medigap plan, and a Part D premium, you will be well over $550/month. Depending upon the extent of benefits, your existing group plan may be approximately the same as this. You should check the totals yourself, but the fact is that the cost sharing under Medigap Plan F will be superior to any group plan. That is because Medigap Plan F has no cost sharing provisions; the premiums are your entire medical cost (except for prescriptions). Remember that while you will be able to opt out of your group plan and into Medicare, that doesn't mean that Medicare will be in its current state, if/when you choose that path. As mentioned earlier, there is speculation that Medigap Plan F may be subject to fundamental change.

There may be tax implications to your selection, depending upon the legal structure of your business. You may be taking a business deduction for the cost of health insurance. You should receive tax or financial counseling before deciding on this important matter. In this particular case, it may be wise to consult your tax advisor.

One word of warning: some insurance companies will not be able to sell certain Medigap plans if you are opting out of group plans. This is above and beyond the "normal" restrictions that occur when a person qualifies for a Special Enrollment Period.

Professional Associations

Doctors, lawyers, accountants, dentists, etc all have professional affiliations of some sort. Within these, there is a decidedly mixed bag. While some organizations are based on a state level, some are national in scope and scale. There can be associations within a profession, like oncologists within physicians. If this is you, you may have been too busy to consider the outside market. You need to consider whether or not the insurance company that sends you the "package deal" is doing so as a commercial endeavor.

> **This happens.**
>
> A professional has been privately insured through his private practice, and continues to work through his 60s. He is eligible and enrolls in Medicare Part A and Part B. In addition, his professional organization offers private health insurance (at group rates), which is more than $300 a month more expensive than Medigap Plan F and a stand-alone prescription drug plan (Medicare Part D). It does so without offering or sending out the professional any information regarding Medigap or the cost sharing arrangement that is available under Medigap. The professional eventually is informed about Medigap and correctly makes the change to Medigap and Part D. It has cost him more than $10,000 in excess premium for coverage that is no better than Medigap and a stand-alone prescription drug plan.
>
> *This happens.*

There is no sense in pointing fingers, and blaming this party or that party. At this point, $10,000 is gone. It doesn't matter how rich you are. $10,000 is a lot of money that could've been otherwise saved or spent (that may be the least controversial statement in this book). *Maximize Your Medicare* is written so you can do something for yourself that others will not. Even professional associations, created to defend its members, can fall woefully short.

Seriously Ill

Those who are seriously ill face difficult choices. When I mean seriously ill, I mean that you have a condition that will not improve through time. Even among those persons, there is a very large difference among the type of illness, and as a result, there are different factors to consider.

If you take a great deal of medications, then you must choose the best stand-alone prescription drug plan (Part D) that you can afford. While the monthly premiums are higher, these plans are more likely to have lower copays for non-generic drugs. In addition, many higher-priced plans will have benefits even inside the coverage gap ("donut hole"). Sometimes, patients take a large number of medications, but do not require visits to the physician often. For example, Alzheimer's patients may, in certain cases, be in a maintenance mode, where relatively few office visits are required. If that is your situation, then the extra dollar should be used for prescription coverage, and not for medical insurance. If you are choosing a Medicare Advantage plan, you should recognize that the prescription benefits within different MA plans can vary, and that can result in a large difference to you.

If you require frequent office visits in order to monitor your situation (for example, Type 1 diabetes), then your situation is slightly different. You will require frequent examinations (eye exam, foot exam) in order to monitor diabetes' progression. In addition, if the situation spins out of control, then the complications are serious, and can potentially require surgical procedures. If this is the case, then it is my view that you require the most comprehensive medical coverage that you can. For you, the Part B Excess may become an issue, because you will most likely have to visit the doctor often, and in bad scenarios, you may be charged more than the Medicare-allowed charge. For this reason, either very comprehensive Medicare Advantage (PPO), or the most comprehensive Medigap policy may be best.

Taking care of these situations is never easy, and we don't have a crystal ball to predict the progression of any given situation. However, it is especially important to think of these scenarios in advance, so that you can respond the situation now, and make the best selection with those scenarios in mind. The reason for this is to preserve the maximum number of options in the future.

Diabetes

There is no easy way to say it: diabetes has reached epidemic proportions in the United States. According the Centers for Disease Control and Prevention (CDC), 25.8 MILLION people in the U.S. have diabetes of some form. Of 10.9 million, aged 65 or older, 26.9% (!!!) had diabetes in 2010. Diabetes is the leading cause of kidney failure, non-traumatic lower limb amputations, and new cases of blindness among adults in the United States.

For people with Type II diabetes, medications are available, and they are very inexpensive. Generics used to treat diabetes are among the cheapest in the market. As long as things do not spin out of control, then it is possible to keep your total health care costs down.

The same cannot be said for those that have Type 1 diabetes. If you do not enroll in a Medigap plan during open enrollment, it will be very difficult to switch into a Medigap policy later. Remember that when the Medigap open enrollment period expires, then you are subject to medical underwriting. Type 1 diabetes frequently disqualifies a new potential enrollee, if the Medigap open enrollment period has expired. That said, if you were leaving a group plan, a certain set of Medigap plans would remain as guaranteed-issue for a period of time. Due the very serious nature of complications caused by Type 1 diabetes, it is very important to obtain the best medical insurance that you can afford.

Prescriptions coverage is also a complicated matter because of the use of insulin. Regarding insulin, Medicare Part B plays a unique role. Needles used for insulin injections are defined as durable medical equipment covered by Medicare Part A. Nowadays, insulin is dispensed via a pen which is part of the prescription; the plastic handle itself is part of the prescription. If you are dependent upon insulin, then you will usually reach the

Medicare Part D coverage gap ("donut hole"). It may be wise to select a Part D plan that has benefits even when in the coverage gap.

End Stage Renal Disease patients and Medicare is quite complicated. In addition to the very high cost of dialysis, the interaction of Medicare, group health insurance, Medicare Advantage and Medigap are very complicated. Here are the simple guidelines. First, Medigap is available for ESRD patients during Medigap open enrollment. Second, Medicare Advantage is, generally speaking, not available for ESRD patients. Third, if you or your spouse work, then you should refer to Chapter 7, and read the section called "Married, Group Coverage, and Medicare: Who Pays First?" The point here is that dialysis is going to be required on a consistent basis with no end. The cost can be enormous over the long run, and it may be wise to divert whatever financial resources are available in order to avoid this out-of-pocket expense.

Chapter 9. Special Topics

How Health Insurance and Life Insurance Are Related

This section is devoted to the interaction between health insurance and life insurance. Health insurance provides coverage for morbidity, which is a state of being ill. Life insurance provides coverage for mortality. When you apply for life insurance, insurance companies may ask you to sign a release, which allows them to access your private health information (PHI). Based on that, insurance companies will record their decision with something called the MIB Group, Inc's database. Both life and health insurance companies belong to this member-owned group. If you have applied for life insurance or health insurance in the past, and you have been refused, then this information will be revealed each time you try to apply for insurance in the future.

For those in the Medicare Initial Enrollment Period, this is no issue. This does not affect your ability to select a Medigap plan of your choosing while in the Medigap open enrollment period. Nor does it affect your ability to select or change a Medicare Advantage (Medicare Part C) plan during the Initial Coverage Election Period (ICEP), Annual Election Period (AEP), or any of the Special Election Periods (SEP). However, your private health information may affect your ability to obtain life insurance.

There are many different types of life insurance. Advertisements can be found everywhere: in the mail, on the radio, and on TV. The two types of life insurance that are most predominant are term and whole (permanent) life.

Term life insurance is easy to understand. You pay premiums until a particular expiry date. Once that expiry date passes, you no longer have life insurance. The insurance company may extend the expiry date, at a different price. That price is generally much, much higher than the one originally paid. There is no cash value established under virtually all term life insurance policies. It is a little known fact that underwriting (i.e. the approval process) can be more difficult under term life insurance than whole life insurance.

Whole life is also easy to understand. You pay premiums, and as long you continue to pay, then the death benefit is paid to the beneficiary that you designate. A cash value is often built, which earns an interest rate that may fluctuate over time, depending on financial markets. If you stop paying premiums, then there are options usually available to you, ranging from a paid-up option to redemption of your cash value. (Note: there can be tax implications to redeeming your cash value, and you should inform yourself of these ramifications beforehand.)

Going forward, this book will deal with whole life insurance. The reason for this is that term insurance is more difficult to obtain than whole life, or permanent, insurance. There is a way to obtain whole life insurance without answering an extensive set of medical questions. You can answer the many fliers that you receive in the mail: they are usually this type of whole life insurance, and will be issued without medical questions. The positive aspect of this is that once the policy has been issued (presuming that you have told the truth about yourself), then it is irrevocable. That means that it remains in place as long as you continue to pay premiums. For this book's purposes, this will be called "Simplified Issue Whole Life Insurance." Insurance companies will have a number of different names for this.

For those without health issues (disease, recent history of surgeries to address ongoing medical problems), a superior alternative exists. This type of insurance is usually not available by simply sending in a flyer in the mail. Generally, you will need to contact an insurance company or agency. There will be specific questions to answer. You may find this cumbersome. For the same price, you would be right. For 30% savings a year, at least, however, it is probably well worth the inconvenience. For this book's purposes, this will be called "Underwritten Whole Life Insurance." Underwritten Whole Life Insurance is at least 30% less expensive than Simplified Issue Life Insurance. The savings in cost of whole life insurance is worth the inconvenience.

The best way to get the best price for whole life insurance is to first obtain Simplified Issue Whole Life Insurance. After it has been issued, then apply for Underwritten Whole Life Insurance. You can then cancel your Simplified Issue Whole Life Insurance. If you do this with the help of an agent, then it is possible to get a refund on your initial Simplified Issue Whole Life Insurance policy. For those without medications, or those without a history of surgical procedures, this is possible. For those with an episode of cancer greater than 10 years ago, this is possible. The standards for approval vary widely, and the prices vary widely.

You will need to draw a careful balance between obtaining the best price, without sending an excessive number of applications. Remember: the MIB is keeping track of this, in order to prevent wrongdoing. In addition, insurance companies may ask you whether you are simultaneously applying for multiple insurance policies.

So why is this explanation given in this book? It is a fair question. The reason is that as Father Time marches on, it is more likely that you will face health issues. I hope not, but that is the reality. With age comes weaker health. Weaker health makes life insurance more difficult to obtain. Older age makes life insurance more expensive to obtain. As you consider health insurance options for the remainder of your life, it is an opportune time to consider final expenses. It is a delicate topic. A complete financial plan, whether you are rich or not, includes life insurance, to prevent being a burden on your remaining family. If your mindset includes thinking about health insurance in order to protect your health and minimize costs, then the same reasoning applies to the best approach to life insurance. Get the best protection that you can reasonably afford, before circumstances, whether within your control or beyond it, change for the worse. If you delay, things will not get easier. This is the central recommendation of the book when it comes to health insurance. Since life insurance also benefits your family as a whole, the same logic can be applied to life insurance.

For those fortunate to have substantial savings, life insurance is an efficient, guaranteed way of passing some of your hard-earned savings to others, whether that is to your extended family, or to your religious organization, or to your favorite charity. It is usually the case that the benefits paid are tax-free. In particular, if you are a female in excellent health, whole life insurance provides a very good return profile compared to other investments that you could leave to beneficiaries.

Home Health Care and Nursing Homes

Taking care of people if they cannot do so for themselves, whether that is due to illness, old age, or a combination of the two, is an issue that is largely unaddressed by our society. It is the proverbial "elephant in the room"; we know it exists and know it is an enormous issue, but we don't discuss it much. The topic is unpleasant at best. Opinions of people vary greatly; some people abhor the thought of being admitted to a nursing home, and others do not. The costs are enormous, particularly if you require skilled nursing care. If you have no savings, then the government will pay for your care, which creates stresses on the already-stressed Social Security system. There are no easy answers for a topic that no one wants to discuss.

Unfortunately, Medicare, or other combinations of Medicare Advantage and/or Medigap, cannot be considered to be long-term care for patients. If you require full-time assistance, or if you require skilled nursing facility care, that is an out-of-pocket expense with substantial potential costs. The costs can add up quickly, and ultimately, they can bankrupt a household if you require an extended stay in a nursing home. You most likely know someone like this. As reported in Forbes magazine, which reported on a study conducted by the Employee Benefit Research Institute (a highly-respected non-profit, non-partisan organization), nursing home residents, on average, lose approximately half (50%) of their savings after six months.

There are insurance solutions. Long-term care insurance, short-term convalescent care insurance, and rides to hospital indemnity plans are three ways that some amounts can be put aside to counter the cost of skilled nursing home facilities.

Advertisements: Treasure or Trash?

A week may not pass by. A month? No way. You have received a mailing which promotes lower health insurance costs. Some are legitimate, and unfortunately, some are not. Turn on the TV, and you get the same thing; commercials about Medicare are everywhere. This is particularly true at the end of every third quarter, and through the end of each calendar year. There are just a few things that you must keep in mind.

First, you should keep all mail from the Centers for Medicare & Medicaid Services (CMS), and mail from The Department of Health and Human Services. It is the official mail from the U.S. Government. The Department of Health and Human Services will send you your Medicare card. If you have a Medicare Advantage or Medigap policy, you should keep all statements from the insurance company that has issued you the policy.

Second, you should not send in an advertisement that offers reduced medication prices if you have any type of group health plan that supplements Medicare. Remember, you cannot be enrolled in two prescription plans that are deemed to be creditable coverage by Medicare. This includes the prescription plan that is embedded in a group plan, or an MAPD plan, as long as your prescription benefits program qualifies as creditable coverage. If you mistakenly send in this type of advertisement that enrolls you in a separate Medicare Part D, then the Medicare system will cancel your enrollment in your employer-sponsored group health plan.

This happens.

Mr. Smith is covered by his retiree group plan, including retiree health benefits. He receives a flyer which suggests that he can save money on prescriptions, and sends it in. Three months later, Mr. Smith requires medical attention, and pulls out the insurance card he has used for years. He finds out that he isn't enrolled in that plan any longer, and he is then responsible for the costs above the amount that Medicare pays. He only has original Medicare. You may know someone that sent in this type of flyer, only to find out that the person has the entire Part A and Part B cost sharing to bear as an out-of-pocket expense.

This happens.

What you need to understand is that advertisements are usually quite vague, and for good reason. The reason is the insurance industry does not want to be accused of being misleading (an insurance company could be subject to regulatory action if this is proven). Therefore, these advertisements are often vague. These advertisements from insurance companies cannot be untrue. Given our litigious society, it is highly doubtful that this will improve anytime soon. The examples presented in this book are

NOT presented in the advertisements. You should read the Disclaimers at the back of this book.

Agents: Angels or Devils?

Agents may or may not offer a valuable service. The nuances of this book should be no surprise to a highly-qualified agent (it is not clear that all agents would reach the same conclusions as this book, given the same set of individual circumstances). However, agents do not necessarily offer every plan available in your area, whether it is Medicare Advantage, or Medigap. Agents may only have permission to offer a limited set of Medigap or Medicare Advantage policies. You, as a consumer, should ask your agent what companies he/she represents. This is actually quite important, as you can see that Chapter 7 is perhaps the most extensive in this book.

Highly qualified agents will be able to quickly and accurately separate fact from fiction. Unqualified agents won't be able to tell you the differences among all the different plans described in this book. In addition, unqualified or inexperienced agents may not be familiar with the impact of very high medical costs on your total savings. Young agents may not have lived through the depression, and may not remember the days of double-digit interest rates.

Additionally, the insurance agents/brokers that deal with your group plan may not have a background in dealing with Medicare. It is very, very important that your agent knows Medicare at least to the level of understanding presented in this book. It is insufficient to only know group health insurance, private health insurance, or auto/homeowner's insurance.

When you have questions regarding your benefits, or controversies about your claims, then a good agent should be able to help. Agents have special access to insurance companies, i.e. they will dial different numbers to ask questions for their clients. If you are the type of person that doesn't like dealing with 1-800 numbers and being put on hold, etc, then a good, attentive agent will be able to help you. They should be experienced in asking the "right" questions, and as a result, a good agent should be able to explain the answers clearly to you.

This happens.

A small business owner is older than 65 but has not yet enrolled in Medicare. His business partner turns 65 next month. They both had been covered using a group health insurance plan. He attempts to *qualify* for an SEP because he is cancelling his group health plan entirely, so that both he and his partner can enroll in Medicare, along with a stand-alone prescription drug plan, and a Medigap plan. He is told that he must wait, and his Medicare Part B will not begin until the next July. The result is that the small business owner, along with his partner, must remain outside the Medicare system, because they do not want to be uninsured.

This happens.

This is totally, completely wrong. He has been misinformed by the Social Security Administration. He can cancel his group health plan, and enroll in Medicare Part B, effective the first of the next month. This is a scary scenario, because the small business owner relied on the information from person representing the government.

There is almost no way that an inexperienced person would have been equipped to defend himself in this situation. Only a person fully confident in the exact rules of Medicare eligibility would have been able to be persistent enough to continue to argue the small business owner's position with the U.S. government, and get him enrolled in Medicare Part B with undue delay or penalty. In this case, an agent's assistance was fully in order. (Yes, it was me.)

One last point about agents: remember that all insurance agents should have a state-sanctioned license. While an agent can make an error, the litigious climate in the U.S. heavily favors people who are Medicare eligible. Very heavily. The CMS sends out people to randomly question agents that are advertising Medicare Advantage plans, to monitor the representations that agents make. Because of that, agents are warned, often, that intentionally misleading statements will subject an agent to sanctions, which can include fines and suspension of his/her license. You, as a consumer, can ask an agent to show you his/her license. There are identification numbers on the license as well. In other words, the idea that an agent is intentionally misinforming you, just to the end of closing a sale, is probably not factually correct. That isn't to say that agents aren't compensated for sales, because they are. However, the downside to telling untruths in order to accomplish this is enormous. It may be that he/she isn't able to explain clearly, but that is on the individual agent, not on agents as a whole. If you are uncomfortable with the advice or answers that you have been given, but require professional help, the solution is simple: find another agent. It's a competitive world, and you will be able to locate one that answers your questions to your satisfaction.

Final Thoughts

The Medicare system isn't perfect, and it is unlikely to become perfect in the future. In fact, it is likely to get worse, as a result of demographics (more people turning 65, who live longer), and the underlying global economy. Turn on the TV for a moment, and the fact is that much of the debate regarding Medicare surrounds the term "Medicare-allowed charge." Medical providers are appealing for more, but the system is financially constrained. The point of this book is not to assign blame, or make judgments about who/what party is right or wrong. There are no proposals regarding how to make the Medicare system better (I am still waiting for the President to ask me). However, it is reasonable to predict that this debate will not be resolved anytime soon.

Medicare isn't meant to be comprehensive health insurance. It would be impossible, and we shouldn't spend too much time in complaining about what it should be and what it should not be. It has nothing to do with politics. Nothing. Even if we all agreed on the priorities and politics of the situation, we can't get around three fundamental facts:

Fact 1. There are an estimated 9,200 turning 65 years old, every day. They are newly eligible for Medicare, and they are living longer. Those numbers will not decline anytime soon.

Fact 2. If your child or grandchild dreams of becoming a medical doctor, he/she is looking at a) $300,000-$500,000 of educational costs, b) extraordinary regulatory and legal risk, c) being a virtual employee of the federal government, and d) no return on investment at all until he/she is 30 years old (when he starts to pay back the debts), but points b) and c) never expire.

Fact 3. If you invested $1000 in a business for 20 years, took large legal and regulatory risks, your products may not work, and even if they do, you can only sell them at your price for 10 years, how much would you want to make a year from that investment? How does $50 a year sound per $1000 invested? Unacceptable, right? Congratulations, now you are a partial owner of Merck, one of the world's largest pharmaceuticals.

If you mix the three facts together, you get an unsavory soup, indeed. In fact, if you think about Fact 2 for a moment, you will be able to understand why it is my opinion that the risk of facing the Part B Excess charge is higher than what is commonly believed. If you had $300,000 of debt, would be in any situation to charge less than the maximum? If that is your grandchild, what would you advise that person? Well, in this case, that person is a medical doctor. Maybe now, it is obvious why it is pointless to even attempt to find an acceptable solution in the near term.

There is a lot of advice out there. Some of it comes from your workplace. Some of it comes from your colleagues from work, your family, or your friends. Sometimes, it will be correct. I hope so. Unfortunately, that is not always the case. The source of misinformation can even come from official personnel.

This is a very difficult topic (i.e. criticizing officials of the government), but one additional point needs to be kept in mind. Employees of the government are human, which means that an individual can be mistaken, and can be motivated by his/her own reasons. *A representative of a non-profit governmental agency should not distribute any marketing material that represents an advertisement for a for-profit company. If this occurs, then help your fellow citizen, and report this to the CMS. Someone is responsible for this, and you are being disserved by receiving this information at that location from unlicensed individuals.* Uninformed people go to government-sponsored agencies, in search for help, and receive erroneous counsel, or receive applications that were not supposed to be distributed in that forum. This is not disputing the good intentions of the people that are trying to help. However, it has been my experience that the information that has been shared is incomplete. That lack of completeness is just what this book is attempting to address.

You should verify these opinions for yourself. Those giving advice, whether they be friends, agents, or your human resources coordinator, may not have complete information. They may have only been through a limited set of circumstances. In other words, their situation may be different from yours. The things that your friends face, you may not. The things that you face, your friends may not. They can be health-related. They can be related to financial flexibility, or your domestic situation. Finally, this book has pointed out that the Medicare system itself may change, and can be expected to change. There are reasons that this book recommends that you take control of the situation.

The forces beyond your control may deteriorate; they have no simple solution, and no easy answers. It doesn't matter what your political affiliation or religion is, there are fewer people paying into the Social Security system, and more people who are eligible for Medicare benefits. You may have devoted your career to an employer, but that employer may no longer be viable, or it may face challenges that must be deemed a higher priority. The lower level of economic activity and the rising cost of benefits for active employees are a couple of the largest of those forces. We can speculate on whom or what is to blame. However, the person that will be affected is you, the Medicare beneficiary.

The choices can be confusing, and it doesn't matter if you are rich or poor. In any financial situation, you can do better by knowing more. Hopefully, this book has given you some more knowledge, so you are not as worried that you don't know something. This book isn't perfect; no individual book can possibly cover every scenario. There are too many exceptions, too many individual cases to possibly address them all in one place. Nevertheless, if you follow these guidelines, and avoid the pitfalls, then you can *Maximize Your Medicare.*

###

Glossary

Activities of Daily Living (ADLs): There are six ADLs. They are eating, bathing, dressing, toileting, transferring (walking), and continence. Long term care insurance may cover a patient if it is documented that he/she cannot conduct three ADLs.

Allowed Charge: The amount Medicare will compensate a medical provider for services rendered. A prescribed amount, called the Allowed Charge. Any amount above the Allowed Charge is called an excess charge.

Annual Election Period (AEP): Also known as the Annual Coordinated Election Period. In 2012, the Annual Election Period (AEP) runs from October 15, 2012 through December 7, 2012. Medicare Advantage and Medicare Part D plans can be changed without restriction during this time.

Assignment of Benefits: The compensation given by the Medicare system to a medical provider. Under a PFFS, the medical provider must accept Medicare's Assignment of Benefits on a case by case basis. Failure by the medical provider to accept the Assignment of Benefits within a PFFS structure will result in no benefits paid from either Medicare or the PFFS plan.

Coinsurance: A percentage of administered services that you, the insured, must pay. For example, if the coinsurance percentage is 20%, then your insurance policy will pay for 80%, and you are responsible for 20%.

Copayments: A fixed dollar amount, which you must pay. For example, stand-alone Part D plans have fixed amounts that you, the insured, must pay, for a given medication.

Cost sharing: The combination of deductibles, coinsurance, and copays under a Medicare Part D, Medicare Advantage, or Medigap plan.

Coverage Gap: Otherwise known as the "donut hole." For 2013, this begins when your total out-of-pocket expenses (deductible plus copays) reach $2930, and lasts until your total out-of-pocket expenses reach $4700.

Creditable Coverage: Qualifies after examination by Medicare. If you have creditable coverage, there will be a certificate, or a page, in your Summary of Benefits that describes your group plan. That certifies that your plan meets certain criteria established by the CMS. If you discontinue coverage (either voluntary or involuntary) under a plan that qualifies as creditable coverage, then you may return to original Medicare, or select Medicare Advantage, Medigap under a Special Election Period (SEP). In addition, you can also select a stand-alone Prescription Drug Plan (Medicare Part D). If your plan loses creditable coverage status, then this is another SEP, and you are entitled to all changes under SEP privileges.

Custodial Care: Care related to Activities of Daily Living (ADLs). Note that this is NOT the same as Skilled Nursing Care. Therefore, it is not covered by original Medicare.

Deductible: A fixed-dollar amount which you must pay *before you receive insurance benefits*. For Medicare Part B, the Part B deductible is $147. This is subject to change by Medicare or your insurance company. The easy way to remember deductible is that *you are first in line* to pay bills up to the Deductible amount. Then, after the Deductible amount is satisfied, you will begin to receive insurance benefits.

Durable Medical Equipment (DME): DME are covered by Medicare Part A, with cost sharing. Medicare Advantage and Medigap plans have cost-sharing arrangements which depend on the plan. Note: needles for insulin injection are part of DME.

End Stage Renal Disease (ESRD): Kidney failure that requires dialysis or transplant. Kidney failure which is not ESRD can occur. ESRD is a specific condition with a percentage failure rate which must be documented for Medicare purposes as well under VA benefits purposes. ESRD patients can purchase Medigap, but are generally not allowed to purchase a Medicare Advantage (MA) plan.

Extra Help program: Federal program which offers financial assistance, to those that qualify, to defray prescription costs, including Part D premiums, deductibles, and copays. Extra help beneficiaries have no restriction in changing their prescription drug plan within a calendar year. Qualification status can be changed by the Social Security Administration (SSA).

Formulary: A list of approved drugs issued by insurance companies. A formulary can change throughout the year, with restrictions imposed by the CMS. Every medical condition must have at least 2 medications in its formulary suitable for use, as determined by the CMS.

General Enrollment Period (Medicare General Enrollment Period): Runs annually from January 1 through March 1 each year, for coverage to begin July 1 of that year.

Health Savings Account (HSA): A bank account, which can best be considered a "Health Expense IRA." In order to open an HSA, you must be enrolled in a High Deductible Health Plan (HDHP). Funds in an HSA can be used to pay for allowable medical expenses, as defined by the U.S. Internal Revenue Service.

HMO (Health Maintenance Organization): An organization that provides medical services via contract with member medical providers and facilities. A primary care physician (PCP) must be selected by the policyholder, and future consultations are approved via referral. If services are received from physicians or facilities, then the HMO will not provide benefits.

Home Health Care: Home health care services are offered by privately-run agencies, sometimes in conjunction with skilled nursing care facilities. Patients receive custodial care at their home on an hourly or daily basis. Medicare does not cover any costs associated with home health care unless it is accompanied by skilled nursing care according to Medicare Part A.

Initial Coverage Election Period (ICEP): Also knows as the Medicare open enrollment period. A seven-month period, with the first date beginning three months prior to your initial eligibility date, and ending on the last day of the third month following the month of your initial eligibility date.

Long Term Care insurance (LTCi): Insurance which covers costs that is used to defray costs when the beneficiary cannot perform 3 ADLs (Activities of Daily Living).

Low Income Subsidy(LIS): See Extra Help program.

Medicare Advantage: Plans that are certified by the CMS on an annual basis. Subject to enrollment rules, with exceptions, called Special Election Periods. May or may not include prescription drug benefits. Restrictions apply with respect to medical provider. Cost sharing terms and conditions are subject to change on an annual basis with the approval of the CMS. These plans must be, on average, superior to original Medicare. Important note: that does not mean that each specific benefit in a particular Medicare Advantage plan must be superior to original Medicare. It means that the plan, as a whole, must be, on average, superior to original Medicare.

Medicare Advantage Disenrollment Period: January 1 – February 14. You can cancel any MA, and return to original Medicare. In addition, you can also purchase a stand-alone prescription drug plan (Medicare Part D) at this time.

Medicare Advantage Prescription Drug (MAPD plan): A type of Medicare Advantage plan. It combines hospital insurance, health insurance, along with prescription drug benefits. It cannot be used with a stand-alone prescription drug plan (PDP, also known as Part D).

Medicare Part A: Hospital insurance as defined by the Centers for Medicare & Medicaid Services (CMS). Includes Skilled Nursing Facility Care, Home Health Care, and Hospice services.

Medicare Part B: Medical insurance as defined by the Centers for Medicare & Medicaid Services (CMS). Includes services administered by physicians.

Medicare Part C: Also known as Medicare Advantage (MA). Medicare Advantage plans include HMOs, PPOs, PFFS, POS, and HMO-SNPs. Medicare Advantage plans replace original Medicare, and insurance carriers process claims (except in the case of POS).

Medicare Part D: Also known as stand-alone prescription drug plans (PDP). Beneficiaries cannot have prescription coverage from two sources. Prescription coverage is subject to a plan formulary. Can be changed annually without restriction during the Annual Election Period (AEP).

Medigap: Also known as Medicare Supplement, Medicare Supplemental Insurance. Plans are labeled with letters A-N.

Military Disability: Complicated system which requires separate application process from Social Security disability. Partial disability categorization is possible. VA-supplied medical insurance and prescription benefits available.

Original Medicare: Medicare Part A and Medicare Part B, in combination, are called original Medicare.

PCP (Primary Care Physician): The physician that you identify if you select a Medicare Advantage HMO. Your PCP must provide a referral if you require services from a specialist.

PFFS (Private Fee For Service): A type of Medicare Advantage plan that requires case-by-case approval by the medical provider. The medical provider must agree to accept the Medicare-allowed charge as full payment. A PFFS is the only Medicare Advantage plan that allows a Medicare beneficiary to also enroll in a stand-alone prescription drug plan (Medicare Part D).

POS (Point of Service): A type of Medicare Advantage plan that has a primary care physician that coordinates in-network referrals. Services received from in-network providers are coded, billed, and coordinated by the PCP. Referrals outside the network are allowed, although the cost sharing arrangement may not be for full payment of services. Services received outside the network must be documented in full by the patient.

PPO (Preferred Provider Organization): A type of Medicare Advantage plan that allows participants to receive services from in-network and out-of-network providers. The number of member providers in a PPO is usually larger than the number of member providers in an HMO, thereby allowing for greater freedom of choice in selecting physicians and facilities. Services received from out-of-network providers have costlier cost sharing terms and conditions than services received from in-network providers.

Short-Term Convalescent Care Insurance: Insurance which can be purchased to provide benefits for skilled nursing home care and, in certain cases, custodial care. Beneficiaries can choose whether or not benefits will include custodial care at his/her home. Limitations exist on the length of time that benefits can be received by the beneficiary.

Skilled Nursing Care: This is a defined term by Medicare. Services must be ordered by a physician, and delivered by a registered nurse (RN) or a licensed practical nurse (LPN). Services must be deemed to be reasonable and necessary for the treatment of illness or injury.

Skilled Nursing Care Facility: Also known as a nursing home. A facility that delivers skilled nursing care. Costs are covered by Medicare Part A only after being admitted inpatient at a hospital for at least 3 days. Long Term Care insurance can be used to defray costs incurred at a skilled nursing care facility.

Social Security Administration (SSA): Governmental agency that determines Medicare eligibility, and Extra Help program qualification.

Social Security Disability Insurance and Supplemental Security Income: Benefits paid to those that require assistance due to disability. Applications for these benefits are difficult to obtain, and legal representation is usually required.

Special Election Period: There are Special Election Periods (SEP), in which you can either return to original Medicare or enroll in a Medicare Advantage (MA) plan. In addition, you can appeal for an SEP as well, if the situation does not fit any of the predetermined categories. A description of the SEPs is listed in Chapter 4.

Summary of Benefits: Document that details cost sharing details with a health insurance policy. You should either a) receive one annually, or b) be able to request this from your insurance company and/or human rights coordinator at an employer. Details will include terms and conditions of enrollment rules, cancellation rules, deductibles, copayments, and premiums. You should keep the most recent copy for reference.

Term Life Insurance: Life insurance that pays a death benefit to the named beneficiary upon the death of the insured, as long as the date of death occurs before or on the date of expiry. If the insured survives beyond the date of expiry, then the insurance ends, and the insured become uncovered. There is usually no cash value associated with Term Life Insurance.

Whole (Permanent) Life Insurance: Life insurance that pays a death benefit to the named beneficiary upon the death of the insured. Coverage does not expire, regardless of attained age of the insured. Premiums may vary, depending upon the terms and conditions of the policy. Whole Life Insurance may build cash value which may accrete based on investment performance.

Bibliography

America's Health Insurance Plans (AHIP). "Trends in Medigap Coverage and Enrollment, 2011." 2012. http://aspe.hhs.gov/health/reports/2011/MedigapPremiums/index.shtml

Andrews, Michelle. 2012, August 20, "Health Law Prompts Review Of Some Medigap Plans; Defining Who Gets Dependent Status," Kaiser Health News, http://www.kaiserhealthnews.org/features/insuring-your-health/2012/health-law-medigap-plans-dependent-status-michelle-andrews-082112.aspx

Graham, Judith. 2012, September 21, "The High Cost of Out-Of-Pocket Expenses," The New York Times, http://newoldage.blogs.nytimes.com/2012/09/21/the-high-cost-of-out-of-pocket-expenses/.

Marchand, Ashley, 2012 September 27, "Stakeholders: Medicare Should Cover Care Received in 'Observation'," California Healthline, http://www.californiahealthline.org/features/2012/stakeholders-medicare-should-cover-care-received-in-observation.aspx

Centers for Disease Control and Prevention, 2011, "2011 National Diabetes Fact Sheet," http://www.cdc.gov/diabetes/pubs/pdf/ndfs_2011.pdf

Centers for Medicare & Medicaid Services, 2012, Medicare and You, http://www.q1medicare.com/pics/ContentPics/MedicareAndYou2012_10050.pdf

Centers for Medicare & Medicaid Services, 2012, Choosing a Medigap Policy: A Guide to Health Insurance for People with Medicare, http://www.medicare.gov/Publications/Pubs/pdf/02110.pdf

Centers for Medicare & Medicaid Services, 2011, "Annual Release of Part 0044 National Average Bid Amount and other Part C & D Bid Related Information," https://www.cms.gov/Medicare/Health-

Plans/MedicareAdvtgSpecRateStats/downloads/PartDandMABen chmarks2012.pdf

Centers for Medicare & Medicaid Services, "Medicare and Other Health Benefits: Your Guide to Who Pays First," http://www.medicare.gov/publications/pubs/pdf/02179.pdf

Centers for Medicare & Medicaid Services, 2012, September, "Medicare & You," (Revised September 2012)"

Centers for Medicare & Medicaid Services, 2011, November, "Understanding Medicare Enrollment Periods (Revised November 2011)" http://www.medicare.gov/publications/pubs/pdf/11219.pdf

Centers for Medicare & Medicaid Services, 2012, "Your Guide to Medicare Special Needs Plans (SNPs)," http://www.medicare.gov/Publications/Pubs/pdf/11302.pdf

Amy S. Kelley, Kathleen McGarry, Sean Fahle, Samuel M. Marshall and Qingling Du, et al., 2012 September, "Out-of-Pocket Spending in the Last Five Years of Life,"

Gleckman, Howard, "A Nursing Home Stay Can Ruin Your Finances," Forbes, 2012 June 22. "http://www.forbes.com/sites/howardgleckman/2012/06/22/a-nursing-home-stay-can-ruin-your-finances/

Karoub, Jeff. 2012, June 14, "Michigan House OKs changes for teachers' retiree health care, leaves retirement plan alone," Crain's Detroit Business, http://www.crainsdetroit.com/article/20120614/FREE/1206199 58/michigan-house-oks-changes-for-teachers-retiree-health-care-leaves-retirement-plan-alone#

Marcum, Diana. 2012, July 12. "Stockton retirees sue to stop city from cutting health benefits," Los Angeles Times, http://articles.latimes.com/2012/jul/12/local/la-me-stockton-retirees-20120712.

Marzilli Ericson, Keith M. 2012, September. "Consumer Inertia and Firm Pricing in the Medicare Part D Prescription Drug Insurance Exchange," NBER Working Paper No. 18359.

National Kidney Foundation®, "ESRD Medicare Guidelines," http://www.kidney.org/professionals/cnsw/pdf/ESRD_medicare_guidelines.pdf

U.S. Census Bureau, Population Bureau, 2008, "U.S. Population Projections."
Veterans Administration, "Veterans Health Benefits Guide," http://www.va.gov/healthbenefits/assets/documents/publications/IB-10-465_veterans_health_benefits_guide_508.pdf

Special Thanks

There are many to thank when considering the completion of this book. In a weird way, their examples have imposed pressure on me to make sure this book is the best that it could be.

First, thanks to my friend Charles Park, who has advised me on important aspects of this book, and more importantly, on life, through his understated example. He has encouraged me to write a book. I doubt this was the topic he had in mind, but nevertheless, his encouragement and friendship has been consistent and unwavering.

Second, I am indebted to Ani Cho Stone (I knew her as Ani Cho). She has been my friend since she was just a few years old. She designed the book cover. Ani Cho Stone is a freelance designer with over 15 years of experience creating digital solutions and building brands online. She collaborates with clients to design websites, online promotions and marketing materials. She has done work for Starbucks and Vitaminwater®, among others. You can learn more about her and see samples of her work at chostone.com. I would recommend her without reservation.

Third, and perhaps most importantly, I want to thank Jeannie Shene of Imlay City, Michigan, who faces formidable challenges of her own. Nevertheless, she has displayed unselfishness, strength, and courage by putting her aging parents' well-being first, without an outward hint of self-pity, although she may have had ample reason. Maybe you are courageous like her. I sincerely hope so.

Disclaimer

All statements in this book are solely the informed opinion of the author. The advice in this book cannot and does not represent financial or investment advice. Such advice requires a deep understanding of a person's specific circumstances. Rather, this book provides examples of situations that are designed to provoke further inquiry by readers to help them understand how to best make Medicare work for them. The opinions stated in this book are not affiliated with, nor endorsed by, the Centers for Medicare and Medicaid Services (CMS).

About the Author

Jae W. Oh, MBA, CLU®, ChFC® is a Chartered Life Underwriter, a Chartered Financial Consultant, and a licensed insurance agent with Bankers Life and Casualty Company, a subsidiary of CNO Financial Group Inc. He has passed the CFP® Certification Exam as administered by the CFP® Board. He has a Master's Degree in Business Administration (MBA) in Accounting and Finance from the University of Chicago (the top-ranked MBA program in the U.S. according to Business Week/Bloomberg, 2nd globally according to The Economist), and a Bachelors of Arts (BA) degree in Economics and Political Science from the University of Michigan, Ann Arbor. Consulting services to individuals, businesses and governments are available. License numbers, accreditations, and references are available upon request. Chartered Life Underwriter (CLU®) and Chartered Financial Consultant (ChFC®) are trademarks of The American College.

CPSIA information can be obtained at www.ICGtesting.com
Printed in the USA
LVOW01s1913110713

342470LV00017B/898/P